TROPICAL DISEASES
A HANDBOOK FOR PRACTITIONERS

OTHER BOOKS BY KEVIN M. CAHILL

Tropical Diseases in Temperate Climates
Health on the Horn of Africa
Clinical Tropical Medicine Vol. I
Clinical Tropical Medicine Vol. II
Medical Advice for the Traveler
The Untapped Resource: Medicine and Diplomacy
Teaching Tropical Medicine

TROPICAL DISEASES
A HANDBOOK FOR PRACTITIONERS

KEVIN M. CAHILL

MD DTM & H (Lond.)

Professor of Tropical Medicine
The Royal College of Surgeons in Ireland
and Director, The Tropical Disease Center, New York City

Technomic Publishing Company, Inc.
265 West State Street
Westport, Connecticut 06880

This edition first published 1976
in the United States of America by
Technomic Publishing Company, Inc.
265 West State Street
Westport, Connecticut 06880

© 1975 Kevin M. Cahill
IBSN 0–87762–199–3
Library of Congress Catalog Card Number 76–11951
Printed in Great Britain by
Heffers Printers Limited, Cambridge

FOR HERSELF

Contents

Foreword   *page* x

Preface   xii

Bibliographical Note   xv

Part I   **PROTOZOAL DISEASES**

1   Malaria   1

2   Amoebiasis   14
     Giardiasis

3   African trypanosomiasis   27

4   American trypanosomiasis (Chagas' disease)   35

5   Visceral leishmaniasis (kala-azar)   42

6   Cutaneous and mucocutaneous leishmaniasis   48

7   Toxoplasmosis   56

Part II   **HELMINTHIC DISEASES**

8   Hookworm   63

9   Filariasis   68

10   Other filarial infections   78
     Onchocerciasis
     Loiasis
     Related infestations

11   Other nematode infections   85
     Enterobiasis
     Ascariasis
     Trichinosis
     Strongyloidiasis
     Trichiasis
     Larva migrans

12 Manson's schistosomiasis   *page* 94
13 Other schistosomal infections   103
      Schistosoma haematobium infections
      Schistosoma japonicum infections
      Rare schistosomal infections
14 Echinococcosis   110
      Alveolar hydatid disease
15 More trematode and cestode infections   117
      Trematode infections
      Cestode infections

Part III   BACTERIAL DISEASES
16 Leprosy   127
17 Cholera   136
18 Plague and bartonellosis   142

Part IV   VIRAL DISEASES
19 Smallpox   146
20 Yellow fever and arbor virus infections   152

Part V   21 Tropical treponemal and rickettsial diseases   160
                   Tropical treponematoses   160
                     Yaws
                     Intermediate forms
                     Pinta
                     Tropical ulcer
                   Tropical rickettsioses   166

Part VI 22 Tropical ophthalmology   170
                   Trachoma
                   Sparganosis
                   Haemoglobinopathies
                   Iatrogenic factors
                   Mechanical factors

Part VII   23   Miscellaneous tropical diseases   *page* 178
                             Effects of heat
                             Kuru
                             Ainhum
                             Tropical sprue

Part VIII   24   Advising the tropical traveller   183

                     Index   192

Foreword

The success which met Professor Cahill's *Tropical Diseases in Temperate Climates* has demanded a new book and it is delightful to be able to write again a Foreword to it. The world, metaphorically speaking, is shrinking. Air travel has brought all peoples within a few hours' journey of one another, and this, together with inexpensive boat travel and the package tour, has within the past decade tremendously increased the numbers travelling to and from the tropics. This increase is an important factor in transferring diseases endemic in one region to others, but a still greater potential hazard is the shortening of transit time brought about by air travel. This has led to the possibility—and the reality—of diseases with short incubation periods being brought to countries where they are rarely seen. Some of these diseases, such as malaria, can be really dangerous and annually cause a significant number of fatalities, others may only be medical curiosities in the places to which they are brought, but all create diagnostic problems. There is also the real danger that some may start epidemics in their new location. Smallpox has already shown how this can happen.

Several epidemics, fortunately small ones, have originated from the rapid transmission from one country to another of persons incubating a disease. Such patients used to develop their diseases while aboard ship, and the health authorities at the port of arrival had ample warning and opportunity to institute measures to limit the spread of infection. But, with air travel, warning of this kind can no longer be expected, and thus probably the greater part of the responsibility for first diagnosing patients with disease has shifted from the immigration health staff to the general practitioner. Now such patients commonly pass immigration officials during the incubation period of their disease, while feeling well, showing no abnormal signs, and not realizing that they have been in contact with infection.

There are, in addition, many diseases with long, silent incubation periods, their duration measured in years rather than days and weeks; schistosomiasis and leprosy fall into this category. They, too, can present difficult diagnostic and public health problems.

It is therefore essential for the properly equipped modern practitioner to have a working knowledge of tropical and other exotic diseases. This book, which has been written with these objectives in mind, is to be welcomed most heartily. In it the essential facts are given on points with which practitioners will wish to be familiar when examining patients from overseas. The book is concise, up to date, and very readable. It should further be of great value to the undergraduate medical student preparing to take his place in the modern medical world. Professor Cahill has performed a very valuable service in writing the book and is to be congratulated on the task which he has accomplished.

A. W. WOODRUFF
MD PhD FRCP DTM & H
London, England

Wellcome Professor of Clinical Tropical Medicine,
The London School of Hygiene and Tropical Medicine
and the Hospital for Tropical Diseases

Preface to Second Edition

This book will reach a medical audience totally different from that for which an earlier volume was written ten years ago.

No longer are tropical diseases considered a rarity in the practice of any physician in a temperate climate, and no longer does the tropical disease specialist seem as a voice crying in the wilderness. In lectures to medical students and physicians throughout the United States, Europe and around the world, one can readily sense the remarkable change from a parochial to an international view. No longer can any physician in America be unaware of the diseases that have come to her shores as a side-effect of the Vietnam conflict. No physician anywhere can afford to ignore the world-wide spread of cholera in the last few years, nor the threat of malaria transmission within his own community by blood transfusions, or among drug addicts as well as in the recent traveller.

This book has been completely revised. Inevitably it remains the view of one physician—tempered by innumerable clinical experiences in the tropics as well as in the temperate climates since my first book appeared more than ten years ago. Other specialists in clinical tropical medicine might approach the problems presented herein in a different form, or emphasize things that I pass over lightly, but my approach reflects the clinical opportunities and problems and responsibilities that I believe will best serve the general physician, who must be aware of tropical infections in differential diagnosis in our modern world. I hope that the excitement, wonder and satisfactions of tropical medicine will be reflected in these pages, for that surely is my intention.

This is not a textbook of parasitology since that is but one of the basic science disciplines on which clinical tropical medicine depends. For too many years tropical medicine, at least in the United States, has been relegated to the parasitology laboratory, taught as an esoteric topic representing the final pre-clinical hurdle for the medical student. This view, always unfortunate, is no longer tenable. The text considers selected parasitic diseases and tries to present relevant information regarding basic life cycles, epidemiology, pathology, clinical manifestations, therapy and prevention. The same approach is followed for selected bacterial, viral, treponemal and rickettsial infections, and for the miscellaneous medical problems that are grouped together as 'tropical' diseases because they flourish in those warm climates where the bulk of the world's population struggle to establish their own identity as new nations in this developing world.

Acknowledgments for *Tropical Diseases in Temperate Climates* were provided in that preface and, where applicable, are tendered here in full measure as well. In addition, I should like to particularly note the generous cooperation of Mr Paul Hamlyn, and the helpful editors and production personnel for their assistance in this new edition.

Finally, I again acknowledge the remarkable woman to whom this book is dedicated, and without whom none of my own efforts would be possible or enjoyable.

KEVIN M. CAHILL

1974

Bibliographical Note

Brief specialist bibliographies will be found at the end of each chapter. In addition, I recommend the following reference books on the general subject of tropical medicine.

Wilcocks, C., and Manson-Bahr, P. E. C. *Manson's Tropical Diseases A Manual of the Diseases of Warm Climates,* 17th edn. London, Baillière Tindall & Cassell, 1972.

Faust, E. C., Russell, P. F., and Jung, R. C. *Clinical Parasitology,* 8th edn. Philadelphia, Lea & Febiger, 1970.

Maegraith, B. G., and Gilles, H. M. *Management and Treatment of Tropical Diseases.* Oxford, Blackwell Scientific Publications, 1971.

Davey, T. H., and Wilson, T. *Control of Disease in the Tropics,* 4th edn. London, H. K. Lewis & Co., 1971.

Marcial-Rojas, R. A. (ed.). *Pathology of Protozoal and Helminthic Diseases.* Baltimore, Williams & Wilkins, 1971.

Ash, J. E., and Spitz, S. *Pathology of Tropical Diseases.* Washington, D.C., American Registry of Pathology, 1968.

I PROTOZOAL DISEASES

1 Malaria

In the vast underdeveloped areas of the tropics—where the majority of the world's population struggle to exist and which, in this jet age, have become the playgrounds of tourists, the arenas of diplomatic conflicts, and the reservoirs for expanding business cartels—malaria rules. No other disease so decimates the infant population, so enfeebles and destroys adults, or serves so well as a reflection of the public health status of an area. Today malaria is, once again, a major clinical challenge in the temperate climates.

The United States, for example, experienced a twenty-five-fold increase in malaria incidence in the late sixties as infected soldiers returned from the Vietnam conflict. Malaria was not seen only in military hospitals. Veterans experienced attacks after discharge to civilian life, and then served as the basis for malaria dissemination in the community through blood transfusions, in the drug addict population, and, occasionally, by direct mosquito transmission since appropriate anopheline vectors exist in many States.

Although numerous malaria control programmes have been successful, there are still some 360 million people living in malarious areas where either there are no eradication schemes or they are at a very early stage of development. The World Health Organization has retreated from its noble, if unrealistic, goal of the global elimination of malaria. Throughout almost all of Africa and many parts of the East, the WHO now stresses 'pre-eradication' efforts, a euphemism that covers establishing basic public health services capable of eventually carrying out the necessary phases in disease control. Furthermore, since the anopheline vectors have increasingly developed resistance to insecticides, since the ecological effects of DDT and other insecticides are just now being seriously investigated and their further broad use is being questioned, and since the parasite has itself developed resistance to many of the drugs currently used in therapy and prevention, the future of malaria eradication is bleak indeed.

Add to the above the present availability of international travel, the growing leisure time, finances and enthusiasm of millions of tourists and businessmen who annually traverse the tropics, and the possibility that malarious relapses may occur years after exposure, and it becomes obvious that malaria will remain a serious threat for generations to come. Since safe and effective therapy is generally available, and since coma, relapsing febrile illnesses, hepatosplenomegaly and nephrosis are only a few of the protean manifestations of malaria, it is essential that this infection be considered in the differential diagnosis of disease in almost any patient who has travelled at any time in a region where malaria is endemic.

Table 1. Life cycle and morphological characteristics of *Plasmodium* parasites causing malaria in human beings

Plasmodium species	Pre-erythro-cytic period (days)	Cycle time (hours)	Persis-tence in man (years)	Characteristics of parasitized red cells	
				Early	Late
P. vivax	8	48	5	Enlarged; Schüffner's dots	12 to 24 merozoites
P. falciparum	4	48	2	Not enlarged; Maurer's clefts; accolé and appliqué forms; multiple in one red blood cell	12 to 24 merozoites; black pigment prominent; schizonts rare in peripheral blood; crescent-shaped gametocytes
P. malariae	13	72	40	Not enlarged; Ziemann's dots; band forms	6 to 12 merozoites; daisyhead form of schizonts
P. ovale	9	48	5	Enlarged; fimbriated ends	6 to 12 merozoites

Pathological features

Four species of parasites of the genus *Plasmodium* commonly cause malaria in human beings. A number of simian malarial infections have been described as unusual zoonotic infections in areas of Southeast Asia where monkeys live in close proximity to man. The four major malarial infections are: *P. vivax* (benign tertian), *P. ovale* (ovale tertian),

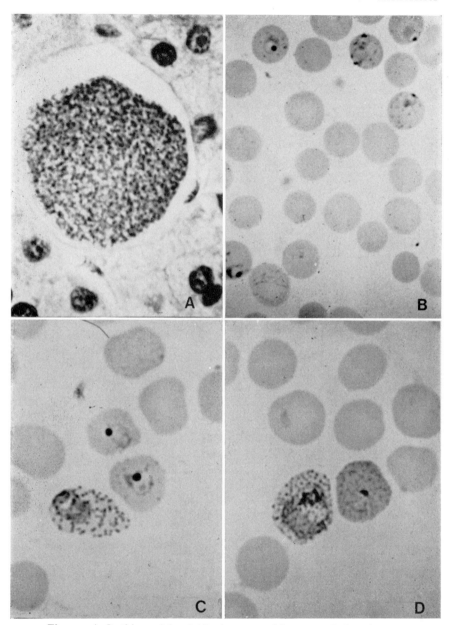

Fig. 1. A–O, thin peripheral blood smears of human malaria. A, pre-erythrocytic schizont in a human liver. B–F, *Plasmodium vivax*: B, early trophozoite or ring forms. C, amoeboid trophozoites and a presegmenting schizont (note prominent Schüffner's dots). D, presegmenter and gametocyte.

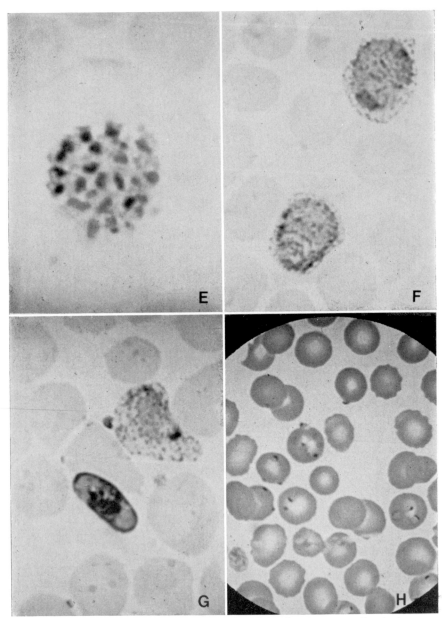

Fig. I *cont.*   E, a mature schizont. F, male and female gametocytes. G, mixed infection with *P. vivax* and *P. falciparum.*   H–J, *P. falciparum*: H, early trophozoites (note multiple infections and appliqué forms).

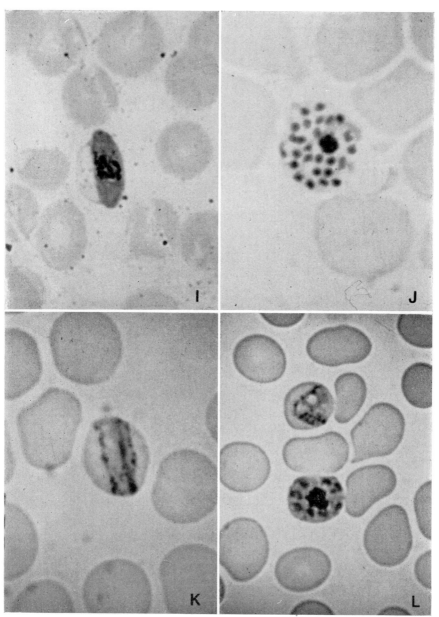

Fig. 1 *cont.* I, crescent-shaped gametocyte. J, a mature schizont, very rarely found in peripheral blood. K–L, *P. malariae*: K, 'band'-form trophozoite. L, 'daisy-head' schizont.

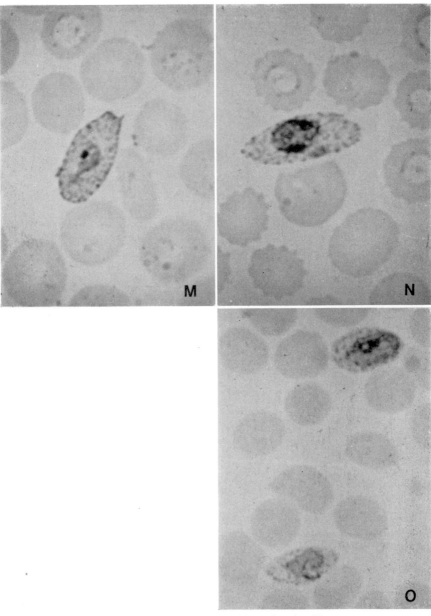

Fig. 1 *cont.* M–O, *P. ovale*: M, amoeboid trophozoite. N, presegmenter. O, gametocyte. Note oval shape and prominent Schüffner's stippling in all stages.

P. falciparum (malignant tertian), and *P. malariae* (quartan). All of these parasites are widely distributed throughout the tropics. Even *P. ovale*, which had formerly been recognized only in certain sections of Africa, has recently been identified in the Philippines, Vietnam and northern South America. Except for the absence of an exoerythrocytic phase in *P. falciparum* infection, the life cycles of these four malarial parasites are similar, with sexual development (sporogony) occurring in appropriate anopheline mosquito hosts and asexual maturation (schizogony) occurring in man. During the act of biting an infected man, Anopheles mosquitoes may ingest male and female gametocytes. The male exflagellates in the insect gut and fertilizes a female parasite. The resulting oocyst then enlarges in the stomach wall for from 7 to 20 days before rupturing into the body cavity, releasing thousands of sporozoites. Those which lodge in the salivary glands may be injected into a new victim when the mosquito bites.

Sporozoites remain in the human bloodstream for less than 1 hour. A few then penetrate parenchymal cells of the liver and undergo pre-erythrocytic schizogony. When the hepatic schizont ruptures 4 to 13 days later (Table 1), merozoites are liberated and can invade new liver tissue or red blood cells. That merozoites from hepatic schizonts of *P. vivax*, *P. ovale* and *P. malariae* can invade new liver cells and thus perpetuate an exoerythrocytic cycle provides an explanation for relapses occurring many years after a single infection. There is no exoerythrocytic phase in *P. falciparum* malaria.

Those pre-erythrocytic merozoites that enter erythrocytes enlarge from a ring form to a trophozoite and, finally, to a schizont (Fig. 1), which, again, can rupture, liberating merozoites that can invade other red blood cells. This cycle of development takes from 48 hours (tertian malaria) to 72 hours (quartan malaria). The severity of pathological changes and clinical manifestations in acute malaria is directly proportional to the percentage of cells parasitized. Since *P. vivax* and *P. ovale* preferentially attack reticulocytes and *P. malariae* attacks aging red cells, less than 10 per cent of erythrocytes are lysed when the schizont ruptures. However, *P. falciparum* invades erythrocytes of all ages, and severe degrees of parasitaemia and resultant anaemia are common in malignant tertian malaria. A few trophozoites do not develop into schizonts but rather into male and female gametocytes which may be ingested by mosquitoes to renew the sexual cycle. The morphological differentiation and the life cycles of *Plasmodium* species are summarized in Table 1 and Figure 1. There are many other distinguishing points, which may be found in a textbook of malariology.

Plasmodium falciparum infection is the only lethal form of malaria. Schizonts (which are rarely found in peripheral blood) block the capillaries of internal organs. Parasitized red cells, malarial pigment and fragments of ruptured erythrocytes adhere to capillary endothelial linings and cause thrombosis, haemorrhage and infarction. This is particularly significant in 'pernicious' *falciparum* infections in which marked pathological changes are seen in the brain (Fig. 2), the heart,

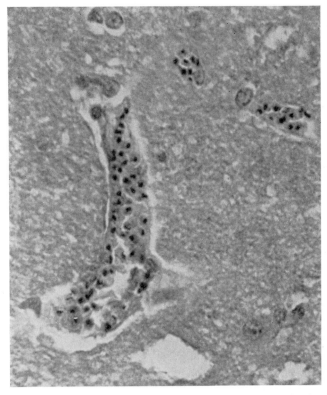

Fig. 2.   Section of the brain from a fatal case of *P. falciparum* malaria, showing blockage of capillaries with pigment and parasites.

or the gastrointestinal tract. Ring or punctate haemorrhages throughout the brain result from parasitic obstruction, and coma is frequently the presenting manifestation of cerebral *falciparum* malaria. Blackwater fever is another fatal manifestation of *falciparum* infection; acute intravascular haemolysis coupled with parasitic blockage of renal capillaries can result in acute tubular necrosis. Rapid haemolytic anaemia can occur, and I have seen patients rupture half their entire red cell mass in

8

6 hours in severe *falciparum* infections. Various consumptive coagulo-
pathies have also been demonstrated in *falciparum* malaria.

In all types of chronic malaria the spleen is almost invariably enlarged.
In acute cases the sudden engorgement with parasitized cells stretches
the capsule, and splenic rupture may result. In chronic cases the
grey-black colour of the spleen from pigment deposition is interspersed
with patchy, white areas of fibrosis from infarctions and perisplenitis
(Fig. 3). The liver also is enlarged and pigmented, with microscopic

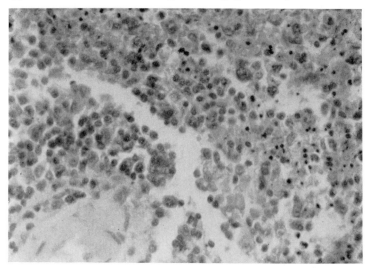

Fig. 3. Splenic biopsy specimen in severe malignant tertian malaria, showing
pigment deposition and fibrosis of white pulp.

evidence of parenchymatous degeneration, centrolobular necrosis,
periportal fibrosis and phagocytosis of pigment and parasites in the
Kupffer's cells. In quartan malaria the pathological changes of nephrosis
may be found.

Clinical features

The initial symptoms of malaria are apparent only after 4 to 13 days
of pre-erythrocytic development in the liver and a further 2 to 3 days
of parasite maturation in the red cell. This long incubation period
increases the probability that unprotected air travellers will present the
first clinical and haematologic evidence of malaria in a temperate zone.
A pathognomonic periodic paroxysm may occur in acute infection with
any of the four species of *Plasmodium* that attack human beings. However, daily temperature spikes are common early in the disease, and it

cannot be emphasized too strongly how rare is the 'textbook' picture of malaria initially present in clinical practice. I have seen acute malaria in the afebrile, in those whose chief complaints were diarrhoea, abdominal pain, cough, and headache. The good clinician must consider malaria whenever there has been exposure.

Usually a febrile pattern evolves that is either tertian (*P. vivax, P. ovale, P. falciparum*) or quartan (*P. malariae*). The paroxysm is similar in all: a cold stage, with severe rigors for from $\frac{1}{2}$ to 1 hour, is followed by a hot stage, of several hours' duration, with rapid temperature rise to 105°F or higher, severe headache, flushed dry skin, nausea, vomiting, and, often, delirium. This is followed by a sweating stage, with profuse perspiration and a feeling of profound exhaustion. Paroxysms generally occur in the late afternoon and may continue for from 3 to 4 weeks. Except in malignant tertian malaria, in which prostration is common, the patient usually feels well in the intervals between paroxysms.

Untreated *P. falciparum* infection either kills or undergoes self-cure within a few months. However, with the other types of malaria, the persistence of exoerythrocytic parasites permits relapses to occur for years (Table 1). In these, the paroxysms are usually less severe, less regular, and, as years pass, they are separated by increasingly longer periods of time.

The complications of acute malaria include herpes labialis (in over 30 per cent of cases), keratitis and, especially in chronic infection, concomitant pneumonitis, cachexia and generalized debilitation. The specific complications of *falciparum* malaria have already been noted.

Diagnosis

To substantiate a diagnosis of malaria, plasmodial parasites must be seen in blood smears or, rarely, in bone marrow, spleen or liver biopsies. With proper staining and persistence, malaria parasites can be demonstrated in all cases of clinical malaria. Positive blood films can be found in patients with acute malaria if repeated blood slides are examined several times a day for from 3 to 4 days. Thick blood films should be examined for the presence of parasites; follow-up thin blood films allow species differentiation. Contrary to a popular practice that I have encountered around the world, blood films should not be taken at the height of the febrile paroxysm. This peak coincides with the rupture of schizonts and the release of merozoites which then appear as small platelet-like dots between red cells. One should examine malaria smears taken every 4 hours throughout the 48- to 72-hour cycle of parasite development within the erythrocyte.

Serological techniques are rapidly becoming established comple-
mentary diagnostic tests in malariology. The indirect haemagglutination and fluorescent antibody tests have been widely and effectively
employed in epidemiological surveys. Refinements in specificity and
sensitivity of these tests will be necessary before they replace standard
microscopy for malaria diagnosis in the general laboratory or, alone,
become the basis for instituting therapy.

Anaemia is usual but is severe only in *P. falciparum* infections.
Leukopenia and thrombocytopenia are common. The serum bilirubin
often is elevated and the urine urobilinogen is raised. In blackwater
fever, haemoglobinuria and marked albuminuria occur. Disappearance
of fever after antimalarial therapy is an inadequate basis for diagnosis.
Periodic pyrexias from many causes are common in the tropics, and a
therapeutic response may be mere coincidence.

Treatment

The word 'cinchona', a synonym for quinine, stems from the legend
that the Countess Chinchon, whose husband was Viceroy in Lima, had
been cured of malaria through the use of 'Peruvian bark' as recommended by the local Indians and, subsequently, had introduced the
medicinal to Europe. This story, though apocryphal, is sufficiently
romantic to have become part of the permanent legend of malaria.
Quinine remained the mainstay of therapy from the mid seventeenth
century until the cinchona plantations of Java fell into Japanese hands
during World War II. This occurred at a time when the number of
soldiers invalided by malaria was ten times greater than the number
lost from action by wounds sustained in battle. Numerous synthetic
antimalarial drugs were produced under the pressure of war and
these revolutionized the therapy and prophylaxis of malaria.

Except in areas where chloroquine resistance is known to exist,
chloroquine is the drug of choice against acute infection with any of
the four *Plasmodium* parasites of man. An oral dose of 1·8 g administered as 600 mg to start, followed by a 300 mg dose 8, 12, 24 and 48
hours later, will completely cure *P. falciparum* infection. If severe
vomiting is a problem, parenteral chloroquine hydrochloride is available. Chloroquine destroys the blood schizonts but does not affect
exoerythrocytic forms. Thus, it may offer 'radical cure' of *P. falciparum*
infection, in which there is no exoerythrocytic cycle, but it will not
prevent relapses in the other three types of malaria. For these, a drug
acting as a tissue schizonticide is essential, and primaquine is recommended. An oral dose of 15 mg daily for 2 weeks is effective. Other
drugs available are listed in Figure 4.

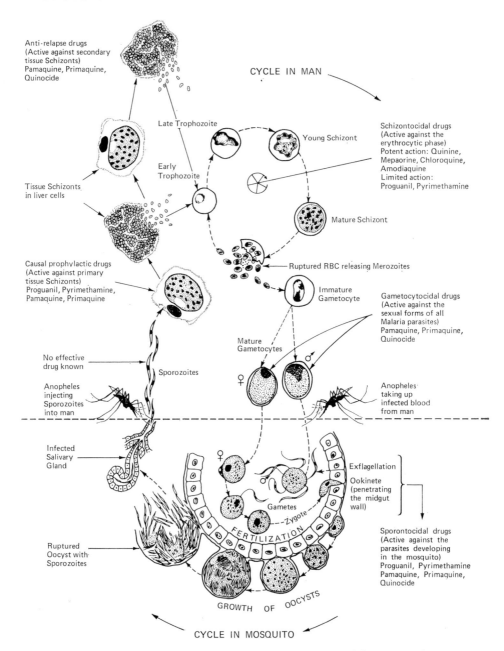

Anti-relapse drugs
(Active against secondary
tissue Schizonts)
Pamaquine, Primaquine,
Quinocide

CYCLE IN MAN

Late Trophozoite

Young Schizont

Schizontocidal drugs
(Active against the
erythrocytic phase)
Potent action: Quinine,
Mepaorine, Chloroquine,
Amodiaquine
Limited action:
Proguanil, Pyrimethamine

Early
Trophozoite

Tissue Schizonts
in liver cells

Mature Schizont

Ruptured RBC releasing Merozoites

Causal prophylactic drugs
(Active against primary
tissue Schizonts)
Proguanil, Pyrimethamine,
Pamaquine, Primaquine

Immature
Gametocyte

Gametocytocidal drugs
(Active against the
sexual forms of all
Malaria parasites)
Pamaquine, Primaquine,
Quinocide

Mature
Gametocytes

No effective
drug known

Sporozoites

Anopheles
injecting
Sporozoites
into man

Anopheles
taking up
infected blood
from man

Infected
Salivary
Gland

Exflagellation

Ookinete
(penetrating
the midgut
wall)

Gametes

Zygote

FERTILIZATION

Sporontocidal drugs
(Active against the
parasites developing
in the mosquito)
Proguanil, Pyrimethamine
Pamaquine, Primaquine,
Quinocide

Ruptured
Oocyst with
Sporozoites

GROWTH OF OOCYSTS

CYCLE IN MOSQUITO

Fig. 4. Classification of antimalarial drugs in relation to different stages in
the life cycle of the parasite.

In areas where chloroquine-resistant *falciparum* malaria occurs—it is currently a major problem throughout Southeast Asia and in small areas of South America—quinine again resumes the first place in therapy, and its rapid administration in a dosage of 10 grains every 8 hours for 7 days may be life-saving. Various combinations of sulphone compounds, pyrimethamine and quinine have been used in the military experience in South Vietnam, but these are trials.

Supportive measures are important in the management of a patient with acute malaria. Hospitalization is advisable but rarely essential in *vivax*, *ovale* and *malariae* infections. Transfusion may be necessary if anaemia is marked. Control of fluid and electrolyte balance is indicated if vomiting or diarrhoea is severe. In addition to being given prompt antimalarial chemotherapy, those with blackwater fever should be managed as are patients with acute tubular necrosis from other causes. The artificial kidney has been used successfully in selected cases. Steroids can be life-saving in cerebral malaria.

Prevention

The tropical traveller can be protected against the danger of malaria by the commonsense use of mosquito netting, long-sleeved shirts, and insect repellents to avoid infection, and by prophylactic medication. As in treatment, so also in prevention, chloroquine is the drug of choice. A weekly dose of 300 mg of the base should be begun on entering a malarious area. Since effective blood levels of chloroquine are attained within hours, it is no longer necessary to commence prophylaxis 10 days before arrival in an infected zone. The drug should be continued for 4 weeks after leaving a malarious area; to prevent relapses from exoerythrocytic forms of *vivax*, *ovale*, or *malariae* infections, primaquine in a daily dosage of 15 mg for 2 weeks is also advisable during that time.

BIBLIOGRAPHY

Cahill, K. (ed.). Malaria—A Symposium. *Bull. N.Y. Acad. Med.* **45**, 997–1101, 1969.
Garnham, P. C. C. *Malaria Parasites and Other Haemosporidia.* Oxford, Blackwell Scientific Publications, 1966.
Peters, W. *Chemotherapy and Drug Resistance in Malaria.* London and New York, Academic Press, 876 pp., 1970.
Russell, P. F. *Man's Mastery of Malaria.* Oxford, 308 pp., 1955.
Maegraeth, B. *Pathological Processes in Malaria and Blackwater Fever.* Oxford, Blackwell, 1948.

2   Amoebiasis

Amoebiasis holds an interesting position in the constellation of 'tropical' diseases in temperate climates. In North America we have experienced some of the greatest water-borne epidemics of invasive amoebiasis known to man, most notably the Chicago epidemic in 1933 and the outbreak at South Bend, Indiana, in 1956. Numerous stool surveys among random populations have shown an incidence ranging from 1 per cent to more than 10 per cent, the vast majority of subjects being asymptomatic. During the first part of this century the causative parasite, *Entamoeba histolytica*, was regarded by most physicians as universally harmful to man. In recent years the pendulum of opinion as to pathogenicity has swung so far that some consider intestinal cysts of *E. histolytica* to be merely commensal protozoa.

Amoebiasis is often, usually unfairly, regarded as the *bête noire* of the traveller, and is probably the most often misdiagnosed ailment of American tourists. Recognition of the aetiological organism requires appropriate laboratory techniques and—equally important—an adequately trained parasitology technician; both are frequently wanting in general hospitals. However, one has to work as a clinician for only a brief period in any of the developing lands to appreciate what great problems amoebic dysentery and intestinal amoebiasis are, and one has to observe but a few patients devastated by amoebiasis to recognize its full potency. This disease is the most common cause of admission to some hospitals in Africa, and the most common cause of death. Tragically, deaths from amoebiasis still occur in New York City— perhaps from lack of awareness that the possibility of the disease exists, for treatment is almost always fully effective if it is provided early enough.

It is obviously crucial to define amoebiasis. What are the criteria for labelling one protozoan, *E. histolytica*, as pathogenic and relieving another of this opprobrium? Are there different strains of *E. histolytica*? What does the organism do in the human body? Can we correlate *in vitro* experiments with our clinical experience? None of these questions can be answered with complete satisfaction today. Yet adequate information is available to permit a working base for the clinician. The clinical prerequisite is an awareness of the possibility, so that amoebiasis will be considered in differential diagnosis.

Pathological features

Entamoeba histolytica is a protozoal organism that can be pathogenic to man. There are at least 6 other amoebas that can parasitize the human intestine but of these (Table 2) only *E. histolytica* is the cause of a significant disease. However, the organism is identified solely on morphological grounds and there are no accurate immunological or culture techniques to distinguish invasive from noninvasive strains. Furthermore, there is evidence that virulent *E. histolytica* amoebas may become avirulent, and vice versa, but there are not, as yet, any procedures to determine why or how or which organisms do this.

Man is infected by ingesting a viable cyst. The cyst wall is resistant to the gastric acidity but disintegrates in the alkaline media of the small bowel, and 8 trophozoites emerge from a single cyst. During active dysentery, trophozoites are found in the stool. However, when faecal movement is slow, the trophozoite reproduces by binary fission, resulting in cysts with from 1 to 4 nuclei in the formed stool. In passed faeces, trophozoites are not infective and are easily destroyed by sun and wind. Cysts, however, may remain viable for weeks. Both may be cultured on a solid, rich, nutritive medium, and amoebic lesions can be produced in experimental animals by intracaecal injection of trophozoites or by the ingestion of cysts.

Trophozoites invade the mucosa of the large bowel both by pseudopodal movement and by secreting cytolytic enzymes, including a proteinase and hyaluronidase, which provide a liquefied medium for spreading themselves. The initial lesion is an erythematous area with a minute central crater. As secondary bacterial inflammation occurs, the ulcer penetrates into the submucosa and extends laterally (Fig. 5), Since the muscularis mucosa is relatively resistant to amoebic invasion, the margins of the lesion pile up, forming the characteristic flask-shaped ulcer with a buttonhole margin. Except in fulminating cases, the lesions of amoebiasis develop slowly enough for reactive proliferation and the formation of thick cicatrization to take place. Therefore, perforation is not common. Intestinal lesions are almost all in the colon, with the small bowel involved only as a direct extension of a caecal infection. The most extensive lesions are found in the caecum, the appendix and the rectosigmoid area.

Extraintestinal amoebiasis is secondary to bowel infection. Although amoebic involvement of almost all organs of the body has been reported, the only sites of statistical significance are the liver and the lungs. Trophozoites are carried from intestinal radicles via the portal venous system to the liver.

Table 2. Minor intestinal protozoa

PARASITE	TROPHOZOITE	CYST	SYMPTOMS	TREATMENT
DIENTAMOEBA FRAGILIS		NOT KNOWN	NONE	NOT INDICATED
ENTAMOEBA COLI			NONE	NOT INDICATED
ENDOLIMAX NANA			NONE	NOT INDICATED
IODAMAEBA BUTSCHLII			NONE	NOT INDICATED
CHILOMASTIX MESNILI			NONE	NOT INDICATED

Organism	Appearance	Symptoms	Treatment
GIARDIA LAMBLIA		OCCASIONAL DIARRHEA AND CHOLECYSTITIS ?STEATTORHEA	MEPACRINE 100 mg t.i.d. x 5 / METRONIDAZOLE 400 mg t.i.d. x 5
TRICHOMONAS HOMINIS		NOT KNOWN	NONE
BALANTIDIUM COLI	*	DIARRHEA DYSENTERY	UNSATISFACTORY ARSENICALS ANTIBIOTICS DIIODOQUINS

0 1 2 3 4 5   1 CM. = 2 MICRONS   *= ½ SIZE

17

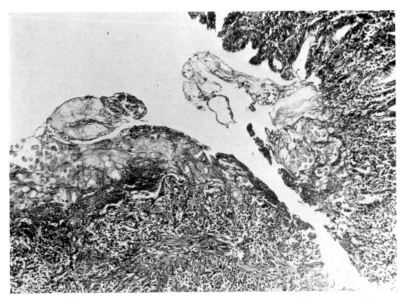

Fig. 5. Amoebic ulcer of the rectosigmoid. *Top*, erosion of the mucosa with involvement and lateral extension in the submucosa. *Bottom*, high-power view of the ulcer margin revealing nests of *Entamoeba histolytica* with leukocytic infiltration.

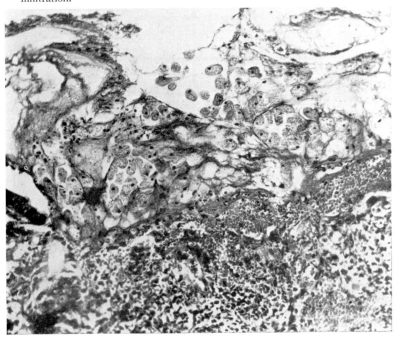

When host resistance is low, and especially if there is hepatic fatty metamorphosis, amoebas invade the liver parenchyma. Cytolysins secreted by the trophozoites provide a liquefied medium for multiplication, and spread and coalescence of abscesses soon occur. The *E. histolytica* organisms are found only in the wall of the abscess, the centre being filled with a necrotic 'anchovy paste' material. The hepatic parenchyma outside the abscess may be normal, and there is no evidence of a true amoebic hepatitis. Over 90 per cent of the abscesses are found in the right lobe of the liver. This has been attributed to haemodynamic streamlining of blood from the heavily involved caecal area.

Pulmonary amoebiasis is due usually to extension from a hepatic abscess and is most frequently localized in the right lower lung field. It occurs in about 15 per cent of those with liver involvement. Bacterial infection is very common, and frank pus is mixed with the characteristic necrotic 'anchovy paste' material. Bronchohepatic and pleural fistulas form in severe cases. Trophozoites of *E. histolytica* may be found in the sputum where the abscess has direct bronchial communication. Direct extension of pulmonary amoebic lesions can also result in pericarditis.

Abscesses of the spleen and brain may follow haematogenous dissemination. Involvement of the skin in the inguinal area is a frequent complication, and cutaneous amoebiasis may follow rupture of hepatic or caecal abscesses.

Clinical features

Less than 10 per cent of patients with intestinal *E. histolytica* infection demonstrate the signs and the symptoms of acute dysentery. Except in recent travellers or in large, water-borne epidemics, the classic syndrome of fever, abdominal cramps, flatulence and copious, bloody bowel movements is rarely detected. Rather, the course of intestinal amoebiasis is commonly slow and insidious. Constipation may be the prevailing symptom; distention and flatulence may be accompanying complaints. Vague symptoms of headache, malaise, insomnia and inability to concentrate may dominate the clinical picture. Pain frequently can be elicited by deep pressure over the sigmoid and the caecal areas. Quite obviously none of these signs or symptoms are specific or pathognomic, and one of the most frequent clinical errors in amoebiasis is to attribute every abdominal complaint to the coincidental presence of *E. histolytica*.

The complications of intestinal amoebiasis are obvious from the discussion on its pathological features. Perforation, although rare

c   19 because of the reactive proliferation in the muscularis, is the most common cause of death in fatal amoebiasis. Appendicitis due to amoebiasis is an important complication, and in the tropics it accounts for approximately a quarter of all cases of acute appendicitis. Surgical treatment in this instance is contraindicated until antiamoebic therapy is administered. In fact, abdominal surgical procedures of any variety in the patient with untreated amoebiasis are associated with appreciable mortality and very high morbidity, since the involved tissue does not retain sutures well. Stool examination should be included among the essential preoperative analyses in any candidate for surgical treatment who has been in the tropics; antiamoebic therapy, if indicated, should precede surgery.

Chronic proliferative cicatrization with resultant bowel strictures and granuloma formation may cause intestinal obstruction. This is most common in the caecal area, where a large granulomatous mass (amoeboma) may be confused with cancer, tuberculosis or actinomycosis. A final significant complication of intestinal amoebiasis is rectal ulceration and fistula formation. Antiamoebic therapy usually will resolve both amoebomas and fistulae.

The signs and the symptoms of amoebic hepatic abscess may appear many years after initial intestinal infection, and two out of three patients give no clear-cut history of previous dysentery. Spiking fevers, chills, weight loss and anorexia are common. The liver is almost invariably enlarged and tender. Jaundice occurs in less than 10 per cent of patients with amoebic liver abscess but is frequent in the small group with left lobe abscesses. Since over 90 per cent of the abscesses are in the right lobe of the liver, the right side of the diaphragm is often elevated, and cough due to diaphragmatic irritation is common.

Pleural and pulmonic amoebiasis usually is due to extension from a liver abscess. Haematogenous spread from intestinal lesions can occur but accounts for less than 10 per cent of pulmonary amoebiasis. There are no clinical features peculiar to amoebic infection in the lungs. Cough, occasionally productive of 'anchovy paste' sputum, chest pain, haemoptysis, the auscultatory signs of pneumonitis, fever and chills are common.

Diagnosis

The definitive diagnosis of intestinal amoebiasis depends on the recognition of the trophozoite or the cyst forms of *E. histolytica*. In acute dysentery this provides no problem at all, since numerous trophozoites can be found in the loose stool. Microscopic examination should be performed whenever possible on fresh, warm specimens. Stool specimens submitted for analysis for amoebiasis are frequently inadequate, often owing to the misguided enthusiasm of the examining physician who has encouraged enemas and purges to obtain a convenient specimen. Many factors can adversely affect the chance of detecting amoebas in the stool; some of them are listed in Table 3. Although

Table 3.   Factors that interfere with parasitological examination of faeces

Factor	Substance
Antidiarrhoeal preparations	Bismuth, kaolin
Radiographic procedures	Barium sulphate
Biologically active drugs	Sulphonamides, antibiotic agents, antiprotozoal drugs, anthelminthic agents
Antacids, laxatives, oils	Magnesium hydroxide
Enemas	Water, soap solution, irritants, hypertonic salt solutions

cysts retain their characteristic appearance in cooled specimens for up to 48 hours, the specimen, if examination must be delayed, should be preserved in a polyvinyl alcohol solution. An iron haematoxylin stain may be used to preserve the smears (Fig. 6). The trophozoite ranges from 15 to 30 microns in size; it has a single, eccentric nucleus, a clear ectoplasmic border, and motile pseudopodia. Ingested red blood cells are frequently noted. The cyst form of the pathogenic larger race measures from 10 to 20 microns. There may be from 1 to 4 nuclei, depending on the maturity of the cyst. The wall is thin, refractile and non-staining.

Various modifications of the direct, iodine-stain, examination enhance the possibility of detecting cysts of *E. histolytica*. The zinc centrifugal flotation technique is commonly employed, and may more than double the diagnostic efficacy of stool examination. Details for this method and other concentration procedures are available in most textbooks of parasitology. The cultivation of trophozoites and cysts of *E. histolytica* on artificial media is possible, but not generally available in most diagnostic laboratories. In patients with liver or pulmonic abscesses one must search for trophozoites in the aspirate, sputum or cavity wall.

Obviously, the services of a parasitologist or a competent technician experienced in stool examination are essential for the recognition of *E. histolytica* and the differentiation between this parasite and other

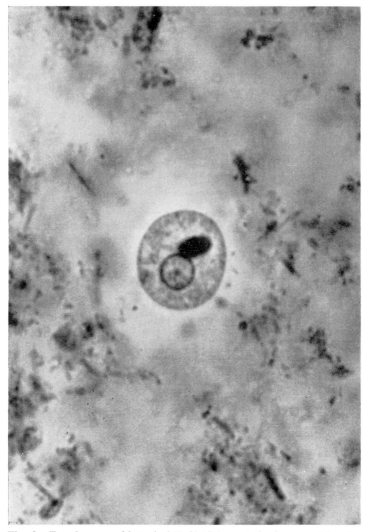

Fig. 6. Faecal smear with typical *E. histolytica* cysts having 4 nuclei and a central chromatin bar.

intestinal protozoa and vegetative faecal forms (Table 2). At least 6 specimens should be examined by direct and concentrating methods before the diagnosis of amoebiasis is eliminated in a suspected case.

In intestinal amoebiasis a sigmoidoscopic examination should always be performed. Since the rectosigmoid area is commonly involved, direct visualization of an ulcer may be possible. Scrapings of the ulcer rim often provide parasitological confirmation of amoebic invasion. Under proper hospital conditions a permanent histological specimen may be obtained by rectal mucosal biopsy (Fig. 5). Barium enemas can reveal multiple mucosal abnormalities, with ulceration in acute cases and thickening in the chronic variety. A narrowed caecum with a funnel-shaped or cone-shaped ileocaecal valve is a characteristic X-ray feature (Fig. 7). An amoeboma will appear as a large caecal tumour.

X-ray studies are also of assistance in the diagnosis of extraintestinal amoebiasis. A scintogram can localize a hepatic abscess. The right side of the diaphragm will be elevated in the majority of right lobe abscesses, and, on fluoroscopic examination, its movement will be limited. Changes of the stomach contour on barium swallow are characteristic of left lobe abscesses.

Percutaneous diagnostic aspiration of a liver abscess is dangerous and should be performed only by an experienced physician in a hospital setting. Prebiopsy coverage with emetine or other amoebicidal drugs is recommended to prevent dissemination of infection along the needle tract. If 'anchovy paste' material is aspirated, therapy should be instituted immediately to avoid spread.

Even after surgical excision, *E. histolytica* are found in only half the patients with hepatic amoebiasis. This low rate is partially due to inadequate examination of the abscess wall where trophozoites lodge. The diagnosis of an amoebic hepatic abscess is in no way influenced by the absence of *E. histolytica* in the stools. In several large series less than 20 per cent of patients with proved amoebic liver abscesses had evidence of current intestinal parasites.

Serology has an important, and ever-growing, role in the diagnosis of amoebiasis. In hepatic abscess and other systemic lesions of invasive amoebiasis, where parasitological confirmation is often impossible or dangerous, serology has become the diagnostic method of choice. Complement fixation, indirect haemagglutination, gel diffusion and fluorescent antibody techniques have all been widely studied, and standardized antigens are now available.

In patients with hepatic amoebiasis, liver function tests are usually normal except for slight derangement in alkaline phosphatase and bromsulphalein (BSP) dye tests.

A 'therapeutic' diagnosis, made by judging clinical improvement to emetine following the failure to demonstrate *E. histolytica* by parasitological or serological methods, is not recommended.

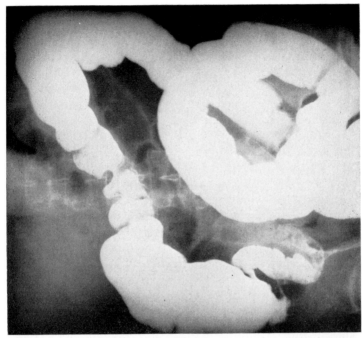

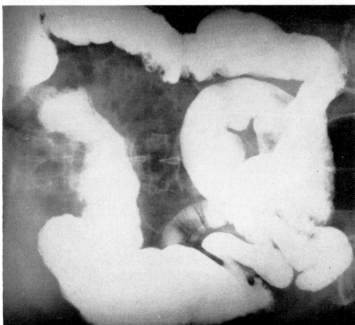

Fig. 7. Barium enema X-rays in a patient with amoebic dysentery. *Left,* before emetine therapy: pretreatment examination reveals diffuse ulceration throughout the large bowel, with narrowing and erosion in the caecum. *Right,* after emetine therapy: post-treatment study shows normal mucosal pattern but persistent narrowing of the caecum.

Treatment

Several dozen compounds are presented by various investigators and pharmaceutical companies as the drug of choice for amoebiasis. It is quite obvious that an ideal amoebicide has not yet been discovered.

Recently metronidazole (Flagyl) has assumed pride of first place in the clinician's armamentarium for both intestinal and hepatic amoebiasis. Depending on the clinical condition, a dosage of 400–800 mg thrice daily for 5 days is frequently curative. The response to Flagyl emphasizes our ignorance regarding geographic and strain differences in *E. histolytica* infection. Although it has been a highly successful therapy in some parts of the world, it has been a failure in others even though the morphological characteristics of the aetiological amoebae are indistinguishable.

For over 50 years the standard therapy for amoebic dysentery and liver abscess was emetine hydrochloride. Despite the danger of cardiac toxicity and the failure to eradicate cystic forms, the judicious use of emetine provides a most effective therapeutic agent for the control of fulminating amoebic dysentery and systemic amoebiasis. The drug must be administered by deep intramuscular injection, since the oral form causes severe nausea and vomiting.

The daily dosage schedule for emetine is 1 mg per kg (maximum, 65 mg) intramuscularly for from 5 to 6 days. This will control the symptoms of acute dysentery, destroy trophozoites, and flatten the fever curve of a patient with hepatic abscess. When the organism cannot be identified, a dramatic response to a trial course of emetine therapy has often been considered to be strong evidence for a diagnosis of amoebiasis. At best, such conclusions are dubious; at worst, tragic. The natural history of several dysenteric disorders is characterized by an abrupt cessation of diarrhoea, and the coincidental administration of emetine not only may be unrelated to the clinical improvement but also may promote a false and dangerous security.

The drug has definite cardiac toxicity; however, severe reactions are rare if the recommended dosage is not exceeded and if vital signs are checked before each injection. If hypotension or tachycardia develops, the drug should be discontinued. Electrocardiograms will show inverted-T waves in early toxicity and conduction defects if emetine is continued. The patient should be at bed rest during the course of therapy. It should not be administered to pregnant women, young children, or patients with cardiac or renal disease.

Emetine does not destroy the intraluminal cyst forms and is of no use in the treatment of chronic or relapsing intestinal amoebiasis. A wide variety of arsenical and hydroxyquinolone drugs have been used for this purpose. Antibiotics are transiently effective; they act by altering the bowel flora, thereby depriving *E. histolytica* organisms of nutriment. However, they do not destroy cysts, and relapses are frequent. Entamide furoate has recently been shown to be an effective agent in the management of ambulatory amoebic patients. One 0·5 g tablet 3 times daily for 10 days will destroy both tissue trophozoites and luminal cysts.

Chloroquine is an effective hepatic amoebicide; but I do not suggest depending solely on it, and usually employ it as a supplemental compound to emetine or metronidazole.

Supportive therapy is, of course, an essential adjunct to the antiamoebic drugs. Strict bed rest is important in the treatment of acute amoebiasis, particularly if emetine is being administered. The diet should include no roughage or bowel irritants. Electrolyte abnormalities secondary to severe dysentery must be corrected lest conduction defects compound the cardiac toxicity of emetine.

The elimination of amoebiasis on a world scale is a public health problem of monumental proportions. Since the disease flourishes where sanitation is poor, eradication is possible only after the education of vast populations in basic hygiene, in the use of properly constructed latrines and water supply systems, and in the elimination of fresh 'night soil' as a fertilizer. Travellers to the tropics should be warned against eating uncooked vegetables and drinking unboiled or untreated water. If they are to reside in the tropics for a time, they should arrange both for periodic stool examinations on their domestic help and for instruction on the importance of post-toilet washing of the hands.

Prevention

I do not believe in so-called intestinal prophylactics as a preventive for diarrhoea. There is no good evidence that any of them are effective, despite the extensive trust that travellers have in compounds such as Enterovioform, and despite the excellent public relations campaigns the drug companies have had on their behalf. Not only are they generally ineffective but they may conceal infections—particularly amoebic infections—until more serious latent effects of these diseases occur. For example, I have seen several cases of amoebic abscess of the liver develop where the patient depended unwisely on intestinal sterilants and where the diagnosis could not be made at an early, treatable stage because these medications interfered with routine stool examination methods.

GIARDIASIS

Giardia lamblia is the only other intestinal protozoan of significance to the clinician. This parasite inhabits the upper intestinal tract causing, particularly in children, a malabsorption-like syndrome. Bowel movements are increased in number, but there is rarely frank, watery diarrhoea, and almost never bloody dysentery. Rather, the stool is bulky, with foul-smelling undigested food particles and fat droplets. An upper gastrointestinal X-ray pattern with clumping of barium and distortion of mucosal folds in the duodenum and jejunum is noted. Small bowel biopsy will not only reveal flattening of intestinal villi but *Giardia* trophozoites can occasionally be seen in the crypts of Lieberkühn. Therapy with metronidazole (Flagyl) or quinacrine hydrochloride (Atrabrine or mepacrine) is effective.

BIBLIOGRAPHY

Cahill, K. (ed.). Amebiasis—A Symposium. *Bull. N.Y. Acad. Med.* **47,** 435–507, 1971.

Shaffer, J. G., Shlaes, W. H., and Rodke, R. A. *Amebiasis: A Biomedical Problem.* Springfield, Ill., Charles C. Thomas, 1965.

Kean, B. H., Gilmore, H. R., Jr, and Van Stone, W. W. Fatal Amebiasis: Report of 148 Fatal Cases from the Armed Forces Institutes of Pathology. *Ann. Intern. Med.* **44,** 831, 1956.

Moore, G., *et al.* Epidemic Giardiasis at a Ski Resort. *New Engl. J. Med.* **281,** 402, 1969.

3 African Trypanosomiasis

Tens of thousands of arable African acres lie fallow today because of the presence of trypanosomes. In tropical areas where malnutrition causes so much infant mortality and adult morbidity, such waste of land is disastrous. For the visitor from a temperate climate, the persistence of sleeping sickness zones may curtail travel plans or even pose a potentially lethal threat. In South and Central America the danger of trypanosomal infection of tourists is less great because of the biting habits and the habitat of the insect vector. In temperate climates the chronic manifestations of this disease are presenting diagnostic challenges with increasing frequency. Throughout wide areas of Latin America, Africa and the Near and the Far East, the dermatological lesions caused by *Leishmania*, a closely related genus of parasites, are deforming thousands each year, and visceral infection with this organism still claims its annual toll.

The trypanosomal and the leishmanial diseases of man differ widely in their geographic distribution, vectors, pathology, clinical manifestations, prognosis and response to treatment. Nonetheless, all of these diseases have certain features in common, since the aetiological parasites are all members of the family Trypanosomatidae. They are all protozoa, and each of them may assume several or all of four developmental forms (Fig. 8): (1) The amastigote (leishmanial form) is an oval organism

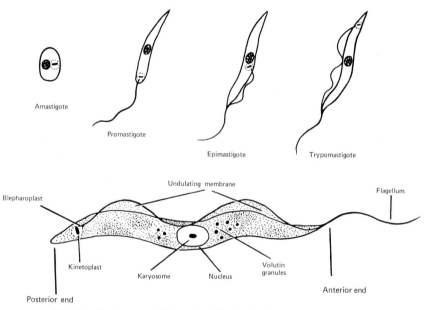

Fig. 8. Developmental forms found in the family Trypanosomatidae.

2 to 5 microns in diameter. It is found in the tissues of patients with all types of leishmaniasis and the American form of trypanosomiasis. The organism has neither an external flagellum nor an undulating membrane. (2) The promastigote (leptomonad form), characterized by an elongated shape 10 to 15 microns in length, a free flagellum but no undulating membrane, and a kinetoplast far anterior to the nucleus, is the infective form found in insect vectors and cultures of leishmaniasis and

is a transitional form in human beings with American trypanosomiasis. (3) The epimastigote (crithidial form) has a kinetoplast just anterior to the nucleus and a free flagellum but no undulating membrane. It is found on culture and in the insect vectors of all human trypanosomal infections. (4) The trypomastigote (trypanosome form) is a motile flagellate form which can be found in the blood, the lymphatic tissue and the cerebrospinal fluid of infected man. In blood films of patients with American trypanosomiasis the monomorphic parasite assumes a 'C' or a 'U' shape and has a prominent posterior kinetoplast. However, in the African types the parasite is polymorphic and may be short and stumpy or long and thin. The position of the nucleus is a distinguishing feature between the two African trypanosomal infections of man.

In Africa two trypanosomes cause human disease. West African sleeping sickness is caused by *Trypanosoma gambiense*, and East African sleeping sickness by *Trypanosoma rhodesiense*. The insect vectors of both diseases are tsetse flies; the West African type is transmitted by riverine *Glossina palpalis* and *G. tachinoides*, while the East African variety is spread primarily by the woodland flies *G. palidipes* and *G. morsitans*. Man is the only reservoir of *T. gambiense*, whereas wild game is the main host of *T. rhodesiense*. Therefore, the habits of the parasites and their vectors determine the epidemiology of human disease. West African trypanosomiasis poses a severe threat to large numbers of people who use rivers for washing, drinking, fishing or transportation. The East African disease primarily affects those wandering in game-inhabited woodland. The presence of an infection can rapidly depopulate a river valley, and the risk of disease prevents vast fertile areas from being cultivated.

Pathological features

The pathological lesions of both types of sleeping sickness are similar, but, since untreated Rhodesian trypanosomiasis is often fatal within a year after infection, gross pathological changes rarely evolve in that form of the disease. More detailed investigations have been made on the Gambian disease, because its untreated victims linger for from 3 to 4 years before death.

At the site of tsetse inoculation, an indurated, erythematous 'chancre' forms in which metacyclic epimastigotes from the insect multiply over a period of 2 to 3 weeks before entering the circulation. At the time of blood-stream dissemination the effects of anaphylaxis may be present, with generalized oedema and erythema. There is a diffuse reticuloendothelial proliferation during the acute stage of infection, with lymphadenopathy prominent, particularly in the Gambian infection.

Myocarditis, keratitis and iridocyclitis are frequent, especially in fulminating Rhodesian infection. Sedimentation rate and globulin levels are elevated, while leukopenia and anaemia are common.

As African trypanosomiasis progresses, the early pathological changes are accentuated, but even more gross alterations occur in the central nervous system. The meninges are covered with a fibrinous exudate, and the gyri are flattened as a result of diffuse cerebral oedema. In the thickened pia arachnoid, mononuclear infiltration around small vessels produces perivascular cuffing (Fig. 9). Diffuse endarteritis is common,

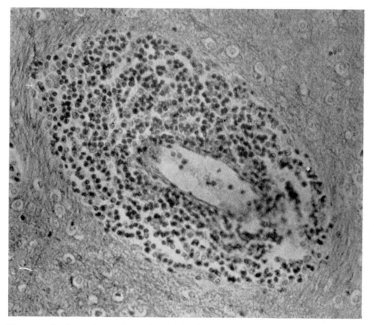

Fig. 9. Perivascular cuffing in the brain of a patient with West African sleeping sickness.

and free trypanosomes have been found in brain tissue. Although they are found infrequently, large, vacuolated and eosinophilic morular cells of Mott are pathognomonic. Pressure, protein and cells—including occasional morular cells—of the cerebrospinal fluid are increased; sugar and chloride levels are low. False positive blood and cerebrospinal fluid Wassermann reactions occur. In the terminal stage, gross wasting and evidence of intercurrent lung or bowel infections are the rule.

Clinical features

The first septicaemic symptoms of African trypanosomiasis appear 2 to 3 weeks after the painful tsetse bite. Relapsing fever of a Pel–Ebstein variety occurs, and concomitant tachycardia persists even during apyrexial periods. In light-skinned persons a transient, circinate,

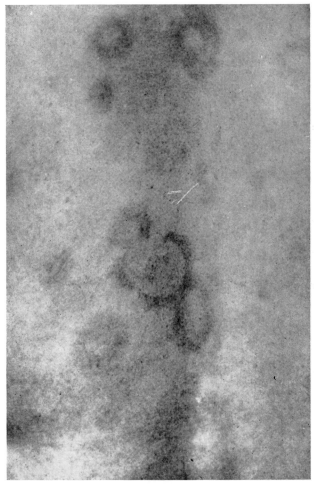

Fig. 10. A circinate, erythematous rash on the back of a light-skinned patient with Rhodesian trypanosomiasis.

erythematous rash may be seen (Fig. 10). Allergic reactions, particularly oedema and asthma, are common. Moderate hepatosplenomegaly can be detected within a few months of infection. Painless lymph node enlargement is generalized, with the posterior cervical chain being most prominent (Winterbottom's sign). With no knowledge of the disease except that its victims died before reaching the market, African slave-traders rejected any captive with this sign. Delayed hyperaesthesia can be elicited, especially over the ulnar nerve (Kerandel's sign). Headache is an early symptom and persists throughout the entire illness. During the acute phase of African trypanosomiasis, the only other manifestations of central nervous system dysfunction are personality changes of fluctuating irritability with lassitude. Despite the appellation 'sleeping sickness', at this stage of the disease insomnia may be marked.

However, as cerebral pathological changes progress, evidence of central nervous system dysfunction dominates the clinical picture. It must again be noted that the victim of Rhodesian sleeping sickness may die before any nervous disorder is apparent. Therefore the gradual Gambian picture is described.

During the waking hours the patient is depressed, confused and apathetic; he complains of severe headache. His speech is slurred, his gait is shuffling, and a tremor of the extremities may develop. However, the most noticeable change is in the ever-increasing somnolence. Sleep may occupy over 20 hours per day, and, although it is possible to arouse the patient for feeding, the lapse back into unconsciousness may occur with the mouth full of food. The nutritional status gradually deteriorates, and the cachectic victim usually dies of intercurrent infection or in a terminal pontine haemorrhage. In rare cases, trypanosomal invasion of the thyroid results in a myxoedematous syndrome (forme bouffée), masking terminal malnutrition.

Diagnosis

The detection of circulating trypomastigotes confirms a diagnosis of either West or East African sleeping sickness. In the Rhodesian disease, parasites are quite readily detectable in the peripheral blood (Fig. 11), and diagnosis usually can be made by thick film examination. However, *T. gambiense* is not as easily found, and accessory sites must often be investigated. Organisms can be sought in aspirated fluid from enlarged lymph nodes, in 'chancre' sites, on marrow and, rarely, in liver or splenic punctures. Parasites or pathognomonic morular cells of Mott may be found in the cerebrospinal fluid; however, they should not be sought in positive *T. rhodesiense* cases without previous drug coverage lest peripheral parasites be introduced into the central nervous system via a traumatic lumbar puncture. Serological techniques are extremely helpful adjuncts in the diagnosis of African trypanosomiasis. Although

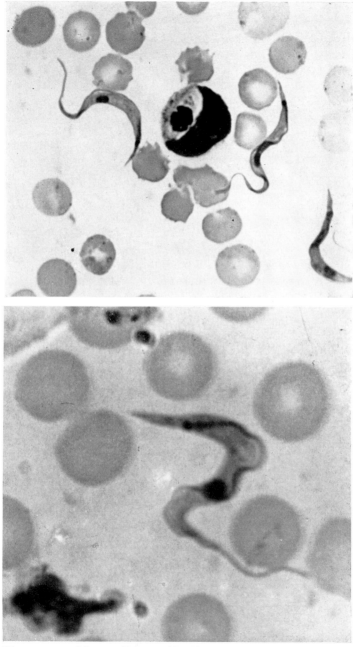

Fig. 11 *top and bottom.* Polymorphic *Trypanosoma gambiense* in peripheral blood of a man with acute West African trypanosomiasis.

it is a nonspecific test, the measurements of IgM levels are very closely correlated with active disease. The fluorescent antibody test is also a useful tool, especially in sleeping sickness surveys. Retrospective diagnosis can be made by demonstrating characteristic cerebral histopathological changes.

Treatment

Specific chemotherapy is almost 100 per cent effective in African trypanosomiasis if administered in adequate dosage early in the disease. Both suramin (Antrypol) and pentamidine isethionate (Lomidine) will eradicate circulating trypanosomes. However, neither drug crosses the blood–brain barrier or can be given intrathecally with safety. If diagnosis is not made till after parasites have invaded the central nervous system, arsenical compounds also must be given.

The drug of choice for early Gambian infection is pentamidine isethionate in an intramuscular dosage of 4 mg per kg daily for 10 days. In early Rhodesian trypanosomiasis, suramin in an intravenous dosage of 1 g in water repeated every 5 days for seven injections is the drug of choice. Hypotension may occur, and it is advisable to begin treatment with a test dose of 0·2 mg. The drug is nephrotoxic, and the urine should be checked for protein and casts prior to each injection. Mel B (Arsobal), a combination of a trivalent arsenical with BAL (British antilewisite), in a single dose of 3·6 mg per kg given slowly intravenously is a satisfactory alternative.

In both East and West African sleeping sickness, once the trypanosomes have entered the central nervous system, arsenicals are essential. Sodium tryparsamide in a weekly intravenous dose of 2 g for 2 to 3 months has been the standard treatment for decades. However, toxic effects, especially primary optic atrophy and encephalopathy, may be marked, and BAL must always be available to enhance excretion. Because of the rapidity of parasitic dissemination in Rhodesian trypanosomiasis, it is advisable to treat East African sleeping sickness patients with Arsobal as well as suramin. An intravenous course of 3·6 mg per kg daily for 4 days may be repeated, if necessary, after a week's rest.

Prevention

Patients from a temperate area visiting a tsetse belt should not receive prophylactic drugs against trypanosomiasis. The toxicity of available drugs far outweighs any dubious benefits the average tourist, whose risk of infection is minimal, might obtain. Inadequate prophylaxis or exposure beyond the 3-month 'protective' period is dangerous, since

34

the early phases of an infection may be masked, becoming evident only when gross pathological changes have occurred in the nervous system. Furthermore, resistant strains of trypanosomes may evolve and cause previously adequate therapeutic regimens to fail. Of course, prophylaxis is of extremely great value for native populations during epidemics.

BIBLIOGRAPHY

Goodwin, L.   The Pathology of African Trypanosomiasis.   *Trans. R. Soc. trop. Med. Hyg.* **64,** 797, 1970.
Duggan, A.   A Survey of Sleeping Sickness in Nigeria from the Earliest Times to the Present Day.   *Trans. R. Soc. trop. Med. Hyg.* **56,** 439, 1962.
Van den Berghe, L., and Lambrecht, F.   The Epidemiology and Control of Human Trypanosomiasis.   *Am. J. trop. Med. Hyg.* **12,** 129, 1963.
Mulligan, H. W. (ed.).   *The African Trypanosomiases.*   Wiley, London, 1970.

4   American Trypanosomiasis (Chagas' Disease)

In every nation of South and Central America and as far north as Maryland in the United States, *Trypanosoma cruzi* exists as a zoonotic parasite. Where climatic conditions are suitable and man lives in close proximity with animal reservoirs and insect vectors, Chagas' disease (human American trypanosomiasis) is common. It is conservatively estimated that some 10 million persons are infected; the majority of cases thus far reported are from Brazil, Venezuela and Argentina, and come mainly from the poor, rural populations who live in thatched-roof or mud-walled hovels infested with *Triatoma* bugs. Although only a few indigenous cases have been reported in the United States, the enormous Latin American immigration, coupled with an increasing awareness of the disease, especially of its chronic manifestations, is responsible for a sharp rise in the number of cases discovered in recent years. With the more frequent use of air transport for farm workers, acute manifestations of the disease may also be expected.

Pathological features

   T. cruzi, the parasite that causes Chagas' disease, is the only one of the human trypanosomes found in all four developmental forms during its life cycle. Trypomastigotes are ingested from the blood of infected man or of a wide variety of animal hosts by the insect vectors, reduviid bugs of the genus *Triatoma*. The parasite alters to an epimastigote stage in the insect stomach but within a month has re-evolved into an infective trypomastigote. Man is infected by contamination of the site of the bug bite with parasite-laden insect faeces. The bite itself may or may not be painful. Because of its habit of attacking the uncovered face, the insect has been ironically referred to either as the 'assassin' or as the 'kissing' bug.

Oedema, inflammation and mononuclear infiltration surround the area of trypanosomal inoculation. Dissemination of the parasite occurs along lymphatic channels and via circulating macrophage cells of the reticuloendothelial system. The parasite multiplies in an amastigote form in reticuloendothelial cells throughout the body. Parenchymatous

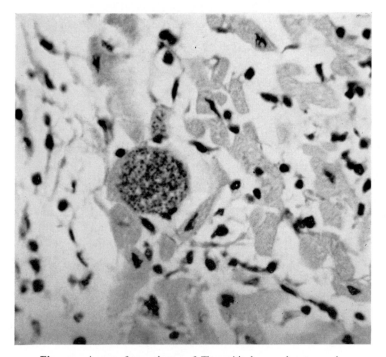

Fig. 12.   A nest of amastigotes of *T. cruzi* in human heart muscle.

degeneration, inflammation and replacement fibrosis in the liver and the spleen may be marked during the acute phase, but even more serious tissue damage occurs in the heart, the intestine and the brain.

Myocardial pathological changes are prominent in both the acute and the chronic phases of Chagas' disease. The rupture of multiplying amastigote 'nests' between cardiac fibres elicits an intense inflammatory reaction (Fig. 12). Endocarditis, myocarditis and pericarditis are common in the early phases, while dilatation and hypertrophy result from progressive destruction of cardiac ganglia and fragmentation, with subsequent hyalinization and fibrosis of myocardial fibres. Similar destruction can be found in skeletal musculature.

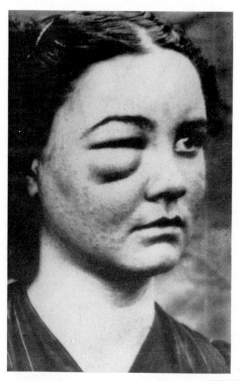

Fig. 13. Unilateral orbital oedema (Romaña's sign), a common initial lesion in Chagas' disease.

Damage to nerve plexuses in the oesophagus and the colon may lead to atony and dilatation of these organs. In acute cases meningoencephalitis may be found. Focal inflammatory reaction and degeneration with granulomatous formation at the site of parasite rupture is often found in the midbrain. Nonspecific inflammatory changes may occur in other organs and in connective tissue.

Clinical features

The earliest evidence of infection is an indurated swelling, or chagoma, appearing within a few hours at the site of the reduviid bite and often persisting for several months. Local lymphangitis with auricular and cervical adenopathy is common. A painless, non-pitting, unilateral facial oedema, especially pronounced about the eye and with an associated conjunctivitis (Romaña's sign), is considered pathognomonic in areas where the disease is endemic (Fig. 13). Nonspecific rashes range from local erythema to diffuse urticarial eruptions with ulceration.

After an incubation period of 1 to 2 weeks, systemic manifestations, which are most severe in children, appear. Fever, which may reach hyperpyrexic levels in infants, begins abruptly and persists for several months, occasionally with a characteristic double-daily spike. Tachycardia is marked and even extends through apyrexial periods in the initial weeks, but a wide range of cardiac arrhythmias may then complicate the clinical picture. Varying degrees of auricular, ventricular and conducting derangements have been described. The heart sounds are usually distant. Diminution of the first sound and a gallop rhythm may be noted in those with acute dilatation and rapid heart failure, and sudden death in these cases is common.

In acute paediatric cases, evidence of central nervous system involvement is sometimes seen, and the very young may present a clinical picture of acute meningoencephalitis. Hepatomegaly can almost always be demonstrated during the acute phase, and the spleen may be palpable. Trypanosomal orchitis and thyroiditis are other well-reported complications of severe infection.

However, it is with chronic Chagas' disease that the clinician in a developed country is most likely to be challenged. Signs of infection may appear after many years of apparent health, and the onset is usually insidious. The clinical patterns may be so protean that only an awareness of the possibility will prevent the unfortunate routine of initial diagnosis being made post mortem. Gradual, progressive heart failure has been recognized as the end-state of the illness since Chagas described the disease in 1909. American trypanosomiasis must be considered in the differential diagnosis of patients, especially young adults, with previously undiagnosed congestive heart failure who have come from or visited an area where the disease is endemic. Suspicion should be heightened if there is cardiomegaly, particularly with dilatation of the right atrium and ventricle, with conduction defects and failure to respond to digitalization.

T. cruzi is also one of the causes of two syndromes long classified as idiopathic, namely, oesophageal achalasia and megacolon, which are common gastrointestinal disorders in Latin America. Clinical, epidemiological and experimental evidence indicates that *T. cruzi* can destroy Meissner's and Auerbach's plexuses and thereby cause atony of the bowel and the oesophagus. Over 90 per cent of patients with alimentary dilatation and hypertrophy in areas of Brazil where Chagas' disease is endemic are known to be infected with *T. cruzi*. In Chagas' mega-oesophagus, dysphagia is progressively incapacitating, regurgitation common, and weight loss marked.

Chronic neurological disease has been described in American trypanosomiasis, but the significance of the association has not yet been proved.

Diagnosis

Laboratory confirmation of a clinical diagnosis of American trypanosomiasis can be accomplished by several highly accurate methods. During the acute febrile phase, circulating trypomastigotes can be seen on stained thick and thin blood films (Fig. 14). A very few additional

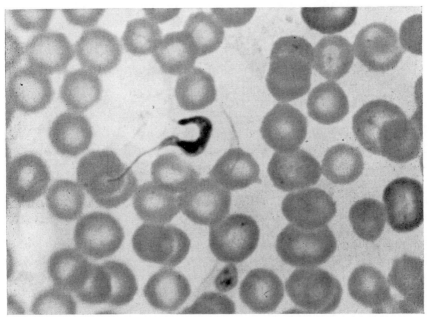

Fig. 14. *T. cruzi* in a thin blood film of a patient with acute American trypanosomiasis. Note the characteristic 'C' or 'U' shape and the prominent posterior kinetoplast.

cases with slight parasitaemia may be detected by concentration techniques, including blood and marrow cultures on N.N.N. (Nicolle–Novy–MacNeal) media, animal inoculation (using puppies, young white rats or a special strain of mice) and xenodiagnosis. In xeno-diagnosis a trypanosome-free reduviid bug is allowed to feed on the suspected patient, and the insect gut is examined 2 to 8 weeks later for the presence of epimastigote forms. The major difficulty with this tech-nique is keeping the insect in the laboratory uninfected with both *T. cruzi* and a common insect protozoan parasite, *T. conorhini*.

Alternative investigations that are useful during the acute phase include a search for trypomastigotes in chagoma fluid or aspirates from enlarged nodes. Muscle biopsy may reveal amastigote nests. An elevated white blood cell count with a dominant lymphocytosis is frequent, and, in those with central nervous system involvement, an increased cell count and a higher protein level are found in the cere-brospinal fluid. Electrocardiographic changes during the acute phase include primary T-wave changes, low-voltage QRS complexes and prolongation of P–R and Q–T intervals. An enlarged cardiac contour can be seen on chest X-rays.

Several serological tests are available for the diagnosis of American trypanosomiasis. A precipitin test is highly accurate during the acute phase of the disease; the more generally available complement-fixation (Machado–Guerreiro) test is highly sensitive and specific in both chronic and acute phases. A brief mention of *T. rangeli*, the other human trypanosome found in South America, suffices, since it is not known to be pathogenic and is morphologically distinct from and does not give serological cross-reaction with *T. cruzi*.

The efficacy of the various diagnostic tests changes when the clinician investigates chronic Chagas' disease. The complement-fixation test and xenodiagnosis become the methods of choice. Blood or tissue fluid examination, animal inoculation and cultures rarely give positive results. However, electrocardiographic changes are often suggestive; a characteristic pattern is: right bundle branch block associated with ischaemic-type T waves and without QRS changes; ventricular extrasystoles; and, often, complete atrioventricular block. Chest X-rays will again demonstrate cardiomegaly, while upper gastrointestinal X-ray series and barium enema examination may reveal a non-specific picture of mega-oesophagus or megacolon.

Treatment

No effective therapy for Chagas' disease is known. A 4-aminoquinolone (Bayer 7602) has trypanocidal effects *in vitro*, but its clinical value is a matter for debate, especially in the chronic stage of the disease, since the drug has no effect on the leishmanial forms in the tissues. The compound 4-aminoquinolone is nephrotoxic and must be administered by painful intramuscular injections. None of the drugs noted in the treatment of African trypanosomiasis is useful against *T. cruzi*. Cardiac failure and arrhythmias do not respond to standard medical regimens. Mechanical dilatation of the oesophagus provides temporary relief in the achalasia of Chagas' disease, and cholinergic drugs and rectosigmoidectomy are of use in managing those with megacolon.

The average traveller visiting a region where Chagas' disease is endemic should be reassured that the possibility of infection is slight, since the triatomid vectors live in thatch or in the mud walls of huts and bite only at night. If such exposure is likely, preliminary spraying with benzine hexachloride (Gammexane) insecticide is advisable; DDT is less effective. Patients should be urged not to sleep on the floor, and beds should be covered with protective netting.

Artificial transmission of American trypanosomiasis through blood transfusion has posed an increasing problem as modern medicine extends in regions where the disease is endemic and emigrants from these regions reach other areas. Whenever possible, a complement-fixation test should be performed on suspected donors. Only negative reactors are acceptable for transfusion supplies.

BIBLIOGRAPHY

Miles, M., and Rouse, J. Chagas's Disease—A Bibliography. *Trop. Dis. Bull.* **67,** Suppl., 1970.

Koberle, F. Chagas' Disease and Chagas' Syndromes: the Pathology of American Trypanosomiasis. *Adv. Parasitol.* **6,** 63, 1968.

Scherb, J., and Arias, L. M. Achalasia of the Esophagus and Chagas' Disease. *Gastroenterology* **43,** 212, 1962.

Woody, N. C., and Woody, H. B. American Trypanosomiasis: I. Clinical and Epidemiologic Background of Chagas' Disease in the United States. *J. Pediat.* **58,** 568, 1961.

5   Visceral Leishmaniasis (Kala-azar)

Only in recent decades has the extent of human leishmaniasis been realized. The visceral form of infection, kala-azar, was formerly believed to be limited to remote rural areas of Africa and Asia. Its incidence has reached epidemic proportions in areas of India and Africa in recent years, and new foci have been discovered in Europe and in South and Central America. The cutaneous and the mucocutaneous forms of leishmaniasis are also broadly distributed. All the leishmanial infections of man, except for the Indian form of kala-azar, are zoonoses but with widely differing animal reservoirs, and all are transmitted to man by the bite of the infective *Phlebotomus* sandfly.

The causative protozoa of all forms of human leishmaniasis are morphologically identical, both as amastigotes (Leishman–Donovan bodies) and as promastigotes, during their life cycle. However, various leishmanial diseases can be distinguished by clinical, epidemiological, histopathological and immunological criteria. Kala-azar—the disease in which the causative organism is *Leishmania donovani*—and its complications will be considered here, while the dermatological diseases will be discussed in the following chapter.

Pathological features

The earliest lesion in kala-azar is a cutaneous nodule, or 'leishmanioma', at the site of the sandfly inoculation. In human volunteer studies—for the initial lesion is observed only occasionally in clinical practice—the maximum size of the nodule, about 2 cm in diameter, is reached in from 1 to 2 weeks after the bite. Promastigotes within the nodule stimulate a granulomatous reaction and a marked round-cell infiltration. The parasites are ingested by circulating macrophages and multiply within these and macrophage cells of the reticuloendothelial (RE) system.

The parasitization and the resultant proliferation of the RE cells is most apparent in the spleen, the liver and the bone marrow. Within 3 months after infection the spleen is palpably enlarged, and, in untreated cases, it may expand progressively to the iliac fossa within a year. Histologically, the splenic architecture is destroyed, with heavily parasitized cells replacing pulp and sinusoids. Although cellular proliferation is marked, inflammation and fibrosis do not occur. Sequestration and destruction of red blood cells increase in direct proportion to the degree of hypersplenia. Thrombosis, with resultant infarction, focal necrosis and perisplenitis, is common.

Hepatic enlargement is less marked, since parasitization and proliferation are limited to the Kupffer's cells. The liver parenchyma can be damaged by pressure atrophy from distended Kupffer's cells, and, in advanced cases, fatty infiltration and fibrosis may be found. Parasitized RE cells replace the normal haematopoietic tissue of the bone marrow and can engorge lymph channels and intestinal villi; in fact, parasites can be demonstrated in every organ of the body.

Anaemia, leukopenia and hypoproteinaemia with hypoalbuminaemia and hypergammaglobulinaemia are characteristic of advanced kala-azar. The anaemia has been attributed both to diminished red cell production from the disrupted bone marrow and to increased destruction of erythrocytes secondary to hypersplenia. The white blood cell count is usually less than 4,000 per cubic millimetre. The granulocytes are depressed, while there is often a relative, and even absolute, mononucleosis. An accompanying thrombocytopenia is found.

Marked serum protein changes have been associated with kala-azar since its discovery and provide the basis for several traditional diagnostic tests. The low albumin levels, often less than 1·5 g per 100 ml (normal level, 4 to 5·6 g per 100 ml), have been attributed to renal and hepatic damage, but without convincing evidence. Alpha, beta and gamma globulins are all elevated in patients with kala-azar, but by far the most significant rise is in the gamma fraction. Electrophoretic studies have shown a specific increase in the 'slow gamma' region as well as the presence of macro- and cryoglobulins.

Clinical features

The initial cutaneous nodule of kala-azar is small and painless, and it is usually not detected. A silent incubation period of from 1 to 4 months follows the sandfly inoculation; prolonged incubation periods of up to 20 years have been reported occasionally. Infants are most commonly affected in the Mediterranean and the American types of kala-azar; both children and adults have the Russian and the African varieties of the disease; and young adults predominate among those with the Indian and the Chinese forms (Table 4). The demonstration that well-nourished, healthy, Americans developed a totally different clinical illness from the same parasite that causes classical kala-azar in the Sudan (Cahill, 1964) emphasized the hitherto unemphasized role of host resistance as a major factor in the eventual presentation

Table 4.   Characteristics of kala-azar in various geographic areas

Type of kala-azar	Age group affected	Glandular enlarge- ment	Animal reservoir	Response to antimony	Occurrence of post-kala-azar dermal leishmaniasis
American	Infants	Yes	Dog, cat, fox	Fair	Rare
African	Children and adults	Yes	Wild rodents	Poor	Occasional
Indian	Adults	No	Man	Excellent	Common
Mediterranean	Infants	Yes	Dog	Fair	Rare
Chinese	Adults	Yes	Dog	Fair	Rare
Russian	Children and adults	No	Dog, jackal	Poor	Rare

of visceral leishmaniasis. In these cases skin manifestations may actually predominate in *L. donovani* infections.

In the 'typical' case, the onset of symptoms is insidious, but it may be sudden and may closely mimic malaria. Fever is usually the earliest manifestation of the disease. A daily, double-remitting pattern, with peaks to 103°F in the late afternoon and the late evening, is character-istic. A concomitant tachycardia persists even during apyrexic periods. Although gastrointestinal disturbances may complicate this early phase, far more often the patient has a striking absence of toxaemia in spite of daily fever, slight hypotension and diffuse disease.

The liver is often palpable by the second month, while splenomegaly may not be detected till the third month. However, the spleen expands progressively and is often grossly enlarged by the time medical treat-ment is sought. In fact, abdominal pain secondary to perisplenitis and anorexia associated with hypersplenism are two of the conditions for which kala-azar victims most frequently first seek medical aid. Ac-companying lymphadenopathy is found in American, African, Mediter-ranean and Chinese visceral leishmaniasis but not in the Indian or the Russian type. In light-skinned patients a grey-black pigmentation may be noted on the forehead and the mid-abdomen. In Bengali the term *kala-azar* means 'black fever'.

As protein and blood cell levels fall, manifestations of chronic kala-azar develop. Oedema and ascites coexist with progressive emaciation and weight loss. Weakness, pallor and ejection heart murmurs of anaemia become evident. Epistaxis and purpura are frequent. With the gradual loss of host resistance mirrored in partial or total agranulo-cytosis, secondary infection flourishes. A particularly common lesion is ulceration of the cheek, or cancrum oris. Pulmonary and intestinal infections are common and are often the immediate cause of death.

The main cutaneous lesion associated with kala-azar is post-kala-azar dermal leishmaniasis. This is a poorly understood lesion that develops several years after apparently successful therapy and is most common in the Indian form of the infection. Amastigotes abound in the skin. Because of the combination of facial nodularity and hypopigmented lesions on the trunk it is often confused with leprosy. The lesions are resistant to diamidines, respond poorly to pentavalent antimonial compounds and, in contrast to visceral lesions, appear to be sensitive to sodium antimony tartrate.

Diagnosis

The demonstration of the causative parasite is necessary for confirmation of a clinical diagnosis. Amastigotes are present in the peripheral blood in Indian kala-azar but are more difficult to detect in the other types. Cultures and animal inoculation will frequently increase, dramatically, evidence of peripheral parasitaemia. Amastigotes can be demonstrated in material from bone marrow, spleen and liver.

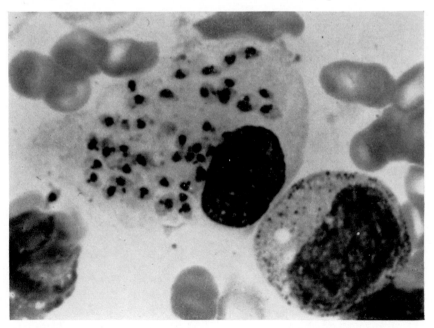

Fig. 15. Bone marrow smear from a patient with visceral leishmaniasis. Numerous amastigotes are found within monocytic cells.

45

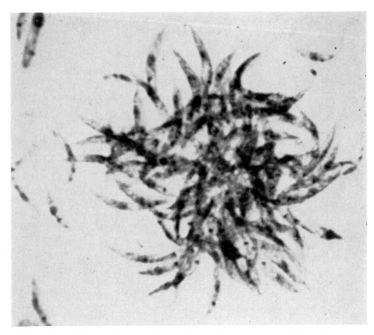

Fig. 16.   Culture of promastigotes from a bone marrow aspirate that was negative on direct smear in a case of Sudanese kala-azar.

Examination of marrow smears is the method of choice (Fig. 15), and culture on N.N.N. media or inoculation into hamsters may reveal scanty infections (Fig. 16). Splenic biopsy has been widely used and is a safe procedure in experienced hands when the spleen is firm. However, it carries risks, and deaths have been reported from splenic rupture or leakage. It should not be employed as an outpatient or field procedure. Although parasites are found in Kupffer's cells, they are far more plentiful in the bone marrow, and liver biopsy is rarely indicated. Complement-fixation tests using as antigens Kedrowsky's acid-fast bacillus (*Mycobacterium phlei*), promastigote cultures, or amastigote suspensions from infected animals have all been widely used, but false negative results occur. An immunofluorescent technique to demonstrate circulating antibodies is also available. The leishmanin skin test is an extremely useful tool, if properly interpreted. It is negative during active kala-azar, but becomes positive after adequate chemotherapy, after self-cure, and during early infection.

Nonspecific supportive evidence includes leukopenia with mono-nucleosis and hypoalbuminaemia with hypergammaglobulinaemia, especially with an increase in the 'slow gamma' region. Several traditional tests for kala-azar are based on the presence of elevated globulins. Both the formol-gel, or formaldehyde, test and Chopra's antimony test are crude turbidity analyses that are helpful in field conditions but are inadequate methods for confirmation in advanced medical centres.

Treatment

Without chemotherapy the majority of patients with kala-azar were thought to die within 2 years of infection. This view had been widely endorsed in texts. However, a major advance has come about through the understanding that host resistance can drastically influence the clinical course, and the evidence from multiple leishmanin skin test programmes that, as with all other infectious diseases, the clinically apparent cases of *L. donovani* disease represent the small tip of the iceberg of aborted, asymptomatic or unrecognized infections.

Two groups of drugs, with varying efficacy against the different geographic types of disease, are used in the treatment of visceral leishmaniasis. Pentavalent antimony compounds (for example, urea stibamine and sodium antimony gluconate) are very effective in the Indian form of the infection, less so in the Mediterranean, African and Russian forms. Urea stibamine in an intravenous dosage of 3 mg per kg of body weight every other day for a total of 14 injections is curative in Indian kala-azar. Sodium antimony gluconate (Pentostam) in an intravenous dosage of 10 mg per kg for 14 days is highly effective in all forms of kala-azar except the African, in which the cure rate rarely exceeds 60 per cent. The parasite is destroyed only toward the end of a course of therapy, and, occasionally, several courses are required. Incomplete or inadequate regimens are dangerous, since they enhance leishmanial resistance.

The diamidines are often necessary for the treatment of African kala-azar and for antimony-resistant patients. However, side-effects with these drugs are common and include hypotension, shock, fever and, occasionally, neuropathies. Pentamidine isethionate is the compound most widely used, and the course comprises intravenous injections of 5 mg per kg of body weight daily for 7 days repeated several times at weekly intervals.

Supportive measures are extremely important in the clinical management of a patient with visceral leishmaniasis. Nutrition must be maintained. Oral hygiene is essential in preventing cancrum oris. Secondary infection must be controlled rapidly by antibiotics, since the neutropenic

47

patient has almost no resistance. Splenectomy for hypersplenia is contraindicated, since the organ resumes almost normal size if drug treatment is successful. If chemotherapy fails, operation does not alter the hopeless prognosis.

Prevention

No prophylactic drug is available. Sandflies can be controlled with DDT or benzene hexachloride insecticide and by repellents, but common mosquito netting is not protective, since the tiny sandfly can easily pass through its mesh. Destruction of animal reservoirs and mass treatment of human hosts, especially those with chronic dermatological lesions, are effective public health control measures.

BIBLIOGRAPHY

Cahill, K.   Field Techniques for the Diagnosis of Kala-azar. *Trans. R. Soc. trop. Med. Hyg.* **64,** 107, 1970.
Cahill, K.   Leishmaniasis in the Sudan Republic: Infection in American Personnel. *Am. J. trop. Med. Hyg.* **13,** 794, 1964.
Manson-Bahr, P. E.   East African Kala-azar. *Trans. R. Soc. trop. Med. Hyg.* **5,** 123, 1959.
Southgate, B., and Oreido, B.   Immunity as a Determinant of Geographical Distribution of Leishmaniasis. *J. trop. Med. Hyg.* **70,** 1, 1967.

6   Cutaneous and Mucocutaneous Leishmaniasis

Leishmanial parasites are responsible for millions of smouldering cutaneous ulcers in Africa, America, the Middle East and the Far East. In the Americas the lesions may spread from the skin to the mucous membranes, resulting in gross facial disfiguration. The usual incubation period of these diseases is from 3 weeks to 3 months, and the clinician must be prepared to diagnose leishmanial sores in recent travellers to or immigrants from regions where the disease is endemic. However, prolonged latent intervals of from 3 to 10 years have been reported. The physician must also be aware of chronic lesions, especially in mucocutaneous leishmaniasis, and should consider these diseases in the differential diagnosis of exposed persons suspected of having skin cancers, lupus vulgaris, fungal infections, leprosy, yaws and syphilis.

Although morphologically indistinguishable, the causative *Leishmania* organisms of the varying cutaneous and mucocutaneous lesions can be separated by epidemiological and clinical criteria. An almost annual variation in the terminology employed to define the aetiological parasites has been confusing, and there is no rational basis to believe that a simple system of disease and parasite nomenclature will be universally accepted in the near future. One classification of cutaneous leishmaniasis is provided in Table 5. It must be remembered that skin

Table 5.   Characteristics of several forms of cutaneous and muco-cutaneous leishmaniasis

Parasite	Usual incubation period (months)	Ecology	Site of lesions	Host reservoir	Response to therapy
L. tropica					
Dry	2 to 12	Town	Face	Man, dog	Good
Wet	< 2	Desert	Limbs	Gerbil	Fair
L. braziliensis	3 to 12	Town, country	Limbs, nose and mouth	Dog, paca	Poor
L. mexicana	< 2	Forest	Ears	Rodents	Good
L. guayansis	< 2	Low mountain	Face, limbs	?	Fair

lesions can occur, and indeed be the only lesions, in *L. donovani* ('visceral') leishmaniasis. Recent immunological investigations indicate that a practical method for laboratory differentiation may soon be available.

CUTANEOUS LEISHMANIASIS

Pathological features. The reservoir of *L. tropica* varies from country to country, with dogs the major host in the Mediterranean, man in the Middle and the Far East, and gerbils or other wild rodents in rural Africa and Asia. The parasite is transmitted to man by the bite of infective species of the *Phlebotomus* sandfly. Two distinct types of cutaneous leishmaniasis, or oriental sore, are recognized: a dry, or urban, variety and a moist, or rural, form. The incubation period of the wet lesion is usually less than 1 month, while the dry sore may not be evident for a year, with latent periods of many years occasionally

49

reported. Although the evolution of lesions in the wet form is much more rapid than in the dry, the pathological changes in the two types are identical.

Promastigotes inoculated subcutaneously by the sandfly are phagocytized and assume an amastigote form within histiocytes. These are found initially in the greatest number in the upper dermis and are surrounded by reactive plasma cells and mononuclear and polymorphonuclear leukocytes. Masses of parasitized histiocytes form tuberculoid nodules in the dermis. As the corium becomes hypertrophied, oedema, perivascular infiltration and small areas of infarction occur. The overlying epidermis is thinned and eventually ulcerates. At this stage acute inflammatory cells invade the ulcer, and secondary infection is common. The centre of the ulcer is often necrotic, and the base of granulation tissue bleeds easily. Parasite multiplication continues at the ulcer periphery, and a zone of inflammation surrounds the crater. Pseudoepitheliomatous hyperplasia with prolongation of the rete pegs results in an elevated edge surrounding the sore. Cicatrization is slow, usually requiring 1 to 2 years, and the final scar is retracted and depigmented and is easily broken down. There are no visceral lesions.

Clinical features. The earliest evidence of infection is a small papule at the site of insect inoculation. This may appear within 2 weeks in the wet type of disease, whereas many months may elapse before its appearance in the dry variety. In the latter, the majority of lesions are on the face, while the exposed limbs are most often affected in wet cutaneous leishmaniasis. Sores are frequently single. As with all infectious diseases, however, there is a spectrum of clinical manifestations, with the most extensive being a severe skin malady easily confused with leprosy. This condition, leishmania tegmenta diffusa, has been most frequently diagnosed in South America and in Ethiopia.

The usual papule enlarges to 2 or 3 cm in diameter over a period of several weeks and is often pruritic and erythematous. Vesiculation occurs, and an oozing, crusted sore develops. If the crust is removed, an oval punched-out ulcer, with elevated, indurated edges, is revealed (Fig. 17). The sore is painless. Small subcutaneous nodules along the draining lymphatic chain, with tender axillary or inguinal adenopathy, are common. Resolution of the lesion is frequently complicated by episodes of bacterial superinfection, and scarring may not be complete for 18 months or more. Generalized symptoms are associated only with bacterial invasion.

Diagnosis. *L. tropica* parasites are demonstrable at the expanding edges of an oriental sore. These should be sought by inserting a needle

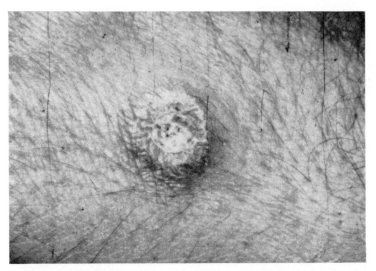

Fig. 17.   Oriental sore with characteristic punched-out appearance.

or a fine pipette through adjacent healthy skin into the ulcer edge, gently rotating the needle for half a minute and aspirating it (Fig. 18). The material should then be examined directly for amastigote forms and, after culture on N.N.N. or diphasic media, for promastigotes. Inoculation of aspirated material into hamsters may occasionally

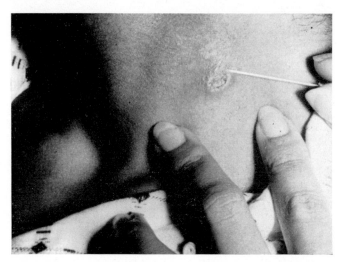

Fig. 18.   Aspirating for amastigotes via the healthy skin adjacent to an oriental sore.

reveal organisms that were indetectable by direct or culture examinations. *Leishmania* organisms rarely are isolated in scrapings from the crater centre. The characteristic histopathological features of oriental sore can be found on biopsy of the ulcer edge, but parasites must be seen in the section before confirmation is possible (Fig. 19).

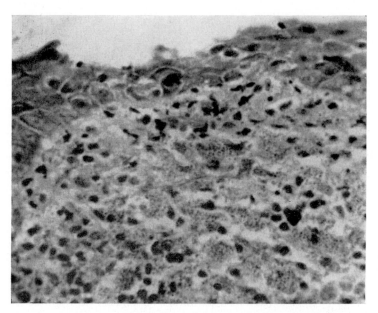

Fig. 19. Multiple amastigotes in the skin of a patient with cutaneous leishmaniasis.

The intradermal test using promastigotes as the antigen can provide serological support for diagnosis but should not, in itself, be the sole basis for chemotherapy. It should, however, re-stimulate the microscopic search for parasites when clinical and epidemiological evidence suggests cutaneous leishmaniasis. A full evaluation of the leishmanin skin test is noted in the bibliography.

Treatment. Intramuscular or intravenous sodium antimony gluconate is necessary to eradicate parasites in lymph nodules and glands. The regimen outlined for kala-azar is recommended. Adequate debridement and sterile dressings are indicated, and antibiotics are required when secondary infection complicates the lesions. Local injections of quinacrine hydrochloride are of dubious value and may, in fact, rupture the limiting ulcer wall. Infection with either *L. donovani* or *L. tropica* confers lasting immunity against future oriental sores.

Despite isolated experimental evidence to the contrary, there appears to be no clinical cross immunity between wet and dry strains of *L. tropica*.

MUCOCUTANEOUS LEISHMANIASIS

Throughout Central and South America a wide variety of leishmanial lesions affect man. The aetiological protozoa are morphologically identical with *L. tropica*, and are also transmitted to man by several *Phlebotomus* species; and the histopathological features are similar to those described for Old World cutaneous leishmaniasis. On clinical and epidemiological grounds a number of distinct types of dermatological disease caused by *Leishmania* can be recognized in the Americas.

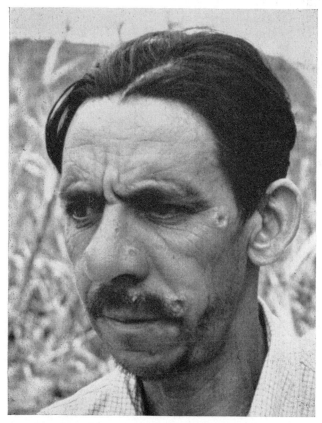

Fig. 20. A patient with several leishmanial ulcers on the face and an enlarged 'tapir' nose: a finding in the early stages of mucocutaneous leishmaniasis.

53

Espundia, or classical mucocutaneous leishmaniasis, existed in Brazil and other South American countries in the pre-Columbian period. Although the facial deformities of its victims have served realistic artists for centuries, the disease has been investigated by clinicians for less than 50 years. *L. braziliensis*, the causative agent of espundia, initially causes a papule and later an ulcer at the site (usually about the face) of sandfly inoculation. Either by direct extension or metastatic spread or by lymphatic dissemination, parasitic invasion of the nasal mucosa occurs in up to 80 per cent of those infected. Granulomatous nodules produce a characteristic 'tapir' nose (Fig. 20) in the early stages of disease, while a related endarteritis may cause perforation of the septum, necrosis and, finally, total destruction. Spread of the lesion to the upper palate, with naso-oral communication and pharyngeal destruction, is rarely found today.

A sylvan leishmanial zoonosis is found in Mexico, Guatemala and Honduras. Those most commonly infected have been adult male chicle-gatherers working and sleeping on moist forest hillsides. The chiclero ulcer is a chronic lesion of the pinna (Fig. 21) without mucosal metastases. There are no generalized symptoms. There is no agreement on

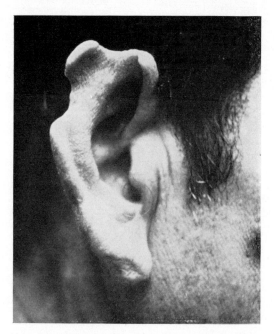

Fig. 21. A chronic chiclero ulcer on the ear of a Mexican chicle-gatherer.

the parasitological terminology of American leishmaniasis, and some investigators refer to the protozoa of chiclero ulcer as *L. tropica mexicana*; others consider *L. braziliensis* responsible for all clinical patterns.

A discrete, ulcerating lesion resembling oriental sore and referred to by the natives as *uta* is common in the mountains of Peru. Mucosal lesions are extremely rare. A chronic, painless ulcer, often associated with lymphadenitis and lymph nodules and with occasional mucosal invasion, is found in Panama, Costa Rica and the Guianas.

Atypical lesions are common in all forms of American leishmaniasis. Non-ulcerating lesions teeming with *Leishmania* parasites can mimic lupus vulgaris, and the verrucous and fungoid eruptions of the disease are often misdiagnosed. Nasal polyps may be the most prominent feature of chronic espundia.

Diagnosis. Again demonstration of the aetiological parasite is the preferred method of diagnosis. Ulcer scrapings, aspirations and biopsies should be examined for amastigotes, and culture and/or animal inoculations may reveal promastigote forms. However, in chronic lesions the search is usually unrewarding, and there is greater dependence on serological evidence in diagnosis of American leishmaniasis than there is in regard to the Old World variety.

Treatment. Espundia, chiclero ulcer and uta are more resistant to chemotherapy than is Old World cutaneous leishmaniasis. Early lesions, especially of the mild Panamanian type, respond to the regimen outlined for oriental sore. However, chronic infections heal slowly, if at all, and the relapse rate is high. Amphotericin B inhibits *Leishmania in vitro* and has been used successfully in man. Pyrimethamine, chloroquine, hydroxystilbamidine and pentamidine have been employed, and each has its protagonists, but none is consistently efficacious.

A lifelong immunity against reinfection by the same strain of the parasite is induced both by cutaneous and by mucocutaneous leishmaniasis. For centuries, natives in zones of Africa and the Middle East where leishmaniasis is endemic have inoculated their children on the buttocks to prevent disfiguring facial scars. Controlled vaccination studies using culture promastigotes as the inoculum are not available. Small-scale projects have shown promise in cutaneous leishmaniasis if vaccination is performed during childhood. The danger of mucosal metastases militates against prophylactic inoculation with live or unaltered *L. braziliensis*.

DDT spraying will destroy sandfly vectors. The delicate *Phlebotomus* is not deterred by the average mosquito net. Protection is best attained by adequate covering of the limbs during the day, and at night by double-net protection of the bed. There are no prophylactic drugs available.

BIBLIOGRAPHY

Cahill, K.   Clinical and Epidemiological Patterns of Leishmaniasis in Africa.   *Trop. geogr. Med.* **29,** 109, 1968.
Cahill, K.   Immunodiagnosis of the Leishmaniases by the Intradermal Skin Test.   *Indian J. Med. Surg,* **36,** 85, 1971.
Adler, S.   Leishmania.   *Adv. Parasitol.* **2,** 35, 1964.
Bryceson, A.   Diffuse Cutaneous Leishmaniasis in Ethiopia.   *Trans. R. Soc. trop. Med. Hyg.* **63,** 708, 1969.

7   Toxoplasmosis

Toxoplasmosis is a parasitic infection that epitomizes many of the features of 'tropical' diseases in temperate climates. It is an affliction of great significance whose clinical incidence is only appreciated as physicians become more aware of the disease. Toxoplasmosis is not limited by geography to the area between the Tropics of Cancer and Capricorn, but has a worldwide distribution. As reports appear substantiating it as a major cause of blindness, as a significant aetiological basis for mental retardation, and as a cause for protean symptoms in the adult ranging from lymphadenopathy to hepatitis and meningitis, toxoplasmosis emerges from the position of an esoteric topic solely interesting the parasitologist to one of enormous interest to all physicians, including obstetricians, paediatricians, ophthalmologists, internists, and neurologists, as well as pathologists and serologists.

Although one stage of the parasite, *Toxoplasma gondii,* was described in 1908, the definitive identification of the infective oocyst form was only completed in the 1970s. The parasite was first recognized in a damaged eye in 1923, but only in recent years has the high incidence of ocular toxoplasmosis been recognized around the world. As the ability of medicine to alter the immune status of the human host develops, toxoplasmosis is emerging as the latest in a long series of iatrogenic diseases; in the patient compromised by immunosuppressive drugs for the therapy of malignancy, toxoplasmosis is a common and serious complication. The disease has, in addition, important economic implications in sheep-raising areas of England, Australia, and New Zealand, and, as with many other 'tropical' infections, has a significance beyond the individual human problem.

Sero-epidemiological studies have clearly demonstrated the frequency of human experience with *T. gondii*; for example, 32 per cent of young women in New York and 84 per cent of those in Paris have antibodies against the infection. Active disease, fortunately, is much less usual, but the impact of both congenital and acquired infections can be great. Nonetheless, the incidence and detection of toxoplasmosis in clinical medicine are almost directly proportional to an awareness of its possibility in differential diagnosis. The very nomenclature of the disease and the parasite is not yet finalized, and the mechanism of infection, transmission, immunity, activation of dormant infection and other basic aspects of the disease are not yet fully understood.

Pathological features

T. gondii is a protozoal parasite that exists in several forms. The proliferative form—occasionally termed a tachyzoite—is an oval-shaped organism 3 to 7 microns long and appears like the merozoite of a malarial parasite. Electron microscopic studies show that there is a complicated system of paired organelles and a double-unit membrane enclosing the parasite. This proliferative form multiplies by endodyogeny and is extremely sensitive to the environment.

Toxoplasma organisms can persist, however, for years in the tissues of hosts as pseudocysts. The cyst, which grows to over 100 microns, is another stage in the life cycle of the parasite. This form is extremely important in human infection since cysts are found in undercooked mutton, beef, and pork, and can withstand the assaults of digestive enzymes as well as the environment. After the cysts are ingested, asexual development of the parasite occurs in the intestine of the cat for approximately 15 days and this stage of gametogony and sporogony is analogous to the development of the malaria parasites.

The oocyst is another form of the parasite; shed in the faeces of the definitive host, cats and other members of the feline family, it is infective for man. Man can be infected by ingesting either the oocysts from cat faeces or the cyst form in infected meat; and the infection can be transmitted transplacentally to the unborn fetus.

The proliferative form of the parasite develops in virtually every organ of the body, and damages cells as they multiply. As *T. gondii* multiplies intracellularly, the affected cells are destroyed and small necrotic foci develop with surrounding hypercellular reaction. Clinically

57

significant lesions are noted primarily in those organs where cell re-
generation does not occur, as in the eye and the brain. When cyst forms
of *T. gondii* rupture, there may be necrosis of surrounding tissue,
partially due to hypersensitivity reaction, and this, again, is of the
greatest significance in those organs where cells do not regenerate. In
congenital infections, cysts also cause damage by obstructing the
cerebral ventricles and the aqueduct of Sylvius, causing further necrosis
of affected tissue.

Human immunity to *Toxoplasma* infection is yet poorly understood
and what factors stimulate the host to respond —or fail to —are not yet
known.

Clinical features

Toxoplasmosis may be either a congenital or an acquired infection.
In the former, the classic combination of intracerebral calcification,
convulsions, hydrocephaly, and chorioretinitis (Fig. 22) is now recognized as the manifestation of severe cases representing the extreme and
relatively rare end of the clinical spectrum. With congenital disease
being more carefully considered, it becomes ever more apparent that
there is a wide range of clinical patterns. Ocular lesions and mental
retardation, for example, may be impossible to determine at birth, and
may become apparent only years after congenital acquisition of
infection.

In Desmonts' classic studies on toxoplasmosis in pregnant women in
Paris and its effect upon their offspring, a number of important observations have been made:

(a) Only those who develop active disease during pregnancy can
transmit the infection to their fetus. The acquisition of infection can be
measured by carefully following *Toxoplasma* titres, and determining
sero-conversion from negative to positive, or by accumulating clinical
data and correlating these with rising *Toxoplasma* serology titres.

(b) Most babies of mothers who acquire toxoplasmosis during pregnancy are not congenitally infected, and only a small percentage of
those that do become infected will actually become symptomatic.

(c) The highest-risk group of babies are those whose mothers became
infected during the first and second trimester of pregnancy. There is
much evidence available, however, that treating mothers promptly
with appropriate antimicrobials will reduce the attack rate on the fetus.

(d) There is no instance known of a woman bearing more than one
child afflicted with congenital toxoplasmosis. This is important to
recognize in advising patients who may wish to become pregnant

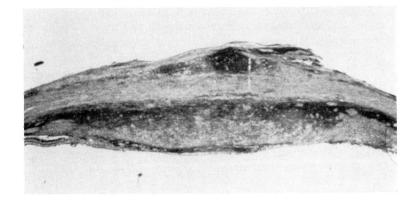

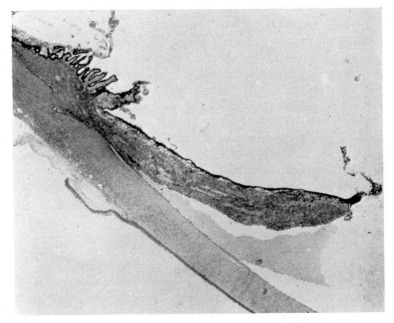

Fig. 22 *top and bottom.*   Chorioretinitis due to toxoplasmosis.

again, and subsequent pregnancies can definitely be considered safe from this point of view.

(e) Although there is question whether maternally acquired toxoplasmosis can cause spontaneous abortion, there is definitely a higher incidence of prematurity in those mothers who have acquired toxoplasmosis during pregnancy.

(f) Analysis of the cerebrospinal fluid in the offspring of mothers who have acquired toxoplasmosis during pregnancy can be prognostically helpful; elevated lymphocyte and protein levels have been demonstrated in apparently asymptomatic offspring.

(g) The offspring of mothers who have acquired toxoplasmosis during pregnancy should be promptly treated with available antimicrobials. In at least one prospective study a significant decrease in the IQ level has been demonstrated in untreated, subclinical congenital toxoplasmosis. There are, however, no control studies to demonstrate, unequivocally, the efficacy of therapy in this group, though available data do indicate benefit.

(h) In congenital toxoplasmosis a wide range of clinical patterns have been demonstrated in addition to the classic lesion noted previously; jaundice secondary to both hepatitis and haemolysis has been recognized, as have pneumonia and encephalitis.

Although the majority of adult patients exposed to *T. gondii* infection do not develop clinical symptoms, the disease must be considered in the differential diagnosis of those with lymphadenopathy, myocarditis, pericarditis, pneumonitis, encephalitis, meningitis, myositis, and arthralgias, nonspecific lymphocytosis, and, of greatest interest, retinochoroiditis and uveitis.

Ocular toxoplasmosis may occur in both congenital and acquired infection. Congenital infections are usually bilateral while the more unusual acquired infections tend to be unilateral. Diagnosis is made by finding a morphologically acceptable lesion in the fundus combined with an elevated *Toxoplasma* serology titre. There is very little correlation between the severity of eye lesions and the serological titre level. Fundal lesions of acute necrotizing *Toxoplasma* retinitis are usually multiple, and appear yellowish to white with fuzzy, indistinct edges and surrounding oedema. Older lesions usually are whitish-grey in colour with heavy pigment deposition, and with distinct margins. These elevated necrotic granulomas are relatively avascular, and that may explain the poor therapeutic results experienced with these cases. The posterior hyaloid membrane may be detached. The optic nerve may be either primarily or secondarily involved.

The differential diagnosis of a necrotizing *Toxoplasma* retinochoroiditis includes tuberculosis, syphilis, histoplasmosis, *Toxocara* infection, and various virus diseases including cytomegalic infection.

The diagnosis of clinical toxoplasmosis may be made by isolation and identification of the organism, serological evidence, or definition of the parasite in histological sections. Aspirates from involved glands and, occasionally, from peripheral blood may yield *Toxoplasma* organisms after intraperitoneal inoculation in laboratory mice.

A wide range of serological tests are available, including the indirect fluorescent antibody (IFA) test, the indirect haemagglutination (IHA) test, the Sabin–Feldman dye test, the complement-fixation test, and the IgM test. In both the IFA and IHA serological procedures, which are the most commonly used tests today, a titre of 1 : 256 suggests either relatively recent exposure or current involvement, while a titre of 1 : 1024 or greater indicates active toxoplasmosis. Meaningful results, however, cannot be based on a single titre and a second specimen should, optimally, be studied after a two-week interval. The IFA test is sensitive and specific, detecting antibodies which appear early in recent and acute infections. The IHA test detects a different system of antibodies which appear later. The dye test, while sensitive and specific, is cumbersome, requiring both living organisms and time-consuming counting procedures. The complement-fixation test, useful in the diagnosis of acute toxoplasmosis, detects antibodies that appear later and disappear earlier than IFA antibodies. The IgM test is a nonspecific procedure, useful for screening, which detects increased levels of IgM resulting from toxoplasmosis infections.

The detection of antibodies in newly born babies establishes the diagnosis of congenital toxoplasmosis, but the wide exposure of humans around the world to infection makes the interpretation of serological studies in this infection difficult for adult acquired disease. Seroconversion from negative to positive, a rising titre, or elevated complement-fixing antibodies are the best evidence of recently acquired, active adult toxoplasmosis.

Treatment

The treatment of toxoplasmosis is an evolving clinical challenge. Adults with systemic infection frequently respond rather dramatically to the classic pyrimethamine–sulphur regimen. A loading dose of 100 to 150 mg of pyrimethamine followed by 25 mg daily for 30 days, combined with triple sulphur compounds in a loading dose of 2 g followed by 1 g four times daily for one month, has been highly successful. It is essential that a white blood cell count be watched weekly since both of these compounds can cause haematological complications. One may administer folinic acid thrice weekly, if necessary, to counter the adverse affects of pyrimethamine. Pyrimethamine and sulphur should not be administered to pregnant women because of the teratogenic effect; Spiramycin would be the current therapeutic choice.

In ocular toxoplasmosis therapeutic results with the pyrimethamine–sulphur regimen are unpredictable and often disappointing. Particularly in chronic progressive inflammatory disease of the fundus, a poor therapeutic response is the rule. In early acute retinochoroiditis the efficacy of therapy is greater; one may add 80 to 100 mg of prednisone daily as an anti-inflammatory agent to the above regimen. It is my opinion that prednisone and other corticosteroids should never be administered alone to patients with toxoplasmosis, but always in combination with antimicrobial agents. Steroids are a two-edged sword, and the recognition that toxoplasmosis has become a major clinical problem in the immunologically compromised host has heightened our awareness of the dangers of this drug.

Newer therapeutic modalities include the drug Spiramycin, an antibiotic derived from *Streptomyces ambofaciens*, and Clindamycin, an antimicrobial that has given very excellent results in experimental ocular toxoplasmosis when administered by retrobulbar injection. Some have suggested the use of laser beam and cryotherapy for treating *Toxoplasma* retinochoroiditis, but these are not yet of proved value. Finally, measures to enhance the immunological ability of the human host may provide the therapeutic course of the future. Some experimental work has indicated the efficacy of BCG administration on this premise.

Prevention

Avoiding oocysts in cat faeces, and infected cysts in undercooked meat, provides the best measure for avoiding infection with *T. gondii*.

BIBLIOGRAPHY

Cahill, K. (ed.)   Toxoplasmosis—A Symposium.   *Bull. N.Y. Acad. Med.*, Vol. 50, 107-239, 1974.

Wolf, A., Cowen, D., and Paige, B.   Human Toxoplasmosis.   *Science, N.Y.* **89,** 226, 1939.

Feldman, H.   Toxoplasmosis. *New Engl. J. Med.* **279,** 1371 and 1431, 1968.

Desmonts, G., and Couvreur, J.   Toxoplasmosis in Pregnancy and its Transmission to the Fetus.   *Bull. N.Y. Acad. Med.*, Vol. 50, 146, 1974.

II HELMINTHIC DISEASES

8 Hookworm

Reviewing his own 40 years of productive laboratory and field investigation in hookworm disease, Stoll noted:

As it was when I first saw it, so it is now, one of the most evil of infections. Not with dramatic pathology as are filariasis or schistosomiasis, but with damage silent and insidious. Now that malaria is being pushed back, hookworm remains *the great infection* of mankind.

He supports this claim by computing the striking facts that the daily blood loss in man from hookworm throughout the world is equivalent to the total exsanguination of $1 \cdot 5$ million people per day and that the total volume of blood transfused annually in the United States represents only half a day's blood loss from the 600-odd million persons around the globe who are infected with hookworm.

Because of the size of the problem it is essential that the physician in temperate climates know of the disease and its treatment. Not only will he be expected to advise travellers to and from areas where the disease is endemic, military personnel visiting torrid zones or industries attempting to cope with the inefficiency secondary to hookworm anaemia, but also he must be prepared to differentiate in temperate regions between hookworm 'infection' and 'disease', to interpret the significance of laboratory reports showing 'positive' findings, and to deal sensibly with infected patients who are now permanent residents in temperate climates. The disease is endemic in every tropical nation, with incidence rates often approaching 90 per cent. Cases are still found in the farm belt in southern United States, and rare outbreaks have been reported from mining areas in Europe, where larval development can take place in warm, moist underground tunnels.

Pathological features

The hookworms that are parasitic in man are, primarily, *Ancylostoma duodenale* (the Old World species) and *Necator americanus* (the New World species). They can be differentiated on morphological characteristics, which are listed in any textbook of parasitology, but it is impractical and unnecessary for the general physician to attempt zoological classification. The life cycle is similar for both parasites.

Eggs deposited by the female worm, which is attached to the human intestinal wall, are passed in the faeces. In the presence of warm (80 to 90°F), moist soil they hatch rhabditiform larvae. After several days of growth and moulting, motile, infective filariform larvae are formed and may remain viable in the soil for from 1 to 2 months. Infection occurs when the human being walks barefoot in contaminated soil, thus giving the larvae the opportunity to burrow through the skin.

This initial invasion causes a pruritic dermatitis which is commonly called toe or ground itch. Oedema and erythema surround the entry point of the larva, and this is followed over a period of 1 to 2 weeks by the formation of a papule and a vesicle. Occasionally, the larvae may migrate intracutaneously, causing a creeping eruption. This picture frequently follows invasion by animal hookworms; the syndrome of 'larva migrans' is discussed in Chapter 11.

After penetrating the skin, the larvae are swept by way of vascular and lymphatic channels to the lungs. Here they migrate through the alveolar wall, causing multiple punctate haemorrhages, and are carried up the tracheobronchial tree and down the oesophagus. During this wandering period, lasting from 2 to 3 weeks, the larvae are enlarging, exsheathing and maturing, so that they are ready and able to attach themselves to the duodenal and the jejunal villi—their destination. Here, with exquisite and devastating efficiency, they exsanguinate the host, copulate and ovulate.

Histological changes in the small bowel are due to a general mechanical irritation as well as to the specific biting and tearing action of the parasite. The teeth may penetrate into the submucosa, with inflammation and eosinophilic infiltration along the tooth marks. The mucosa becomes thin and may ulcerate. Submucosal haemorrhage and cicatrization are common. Intestinal mucosal changes of the malabsorption state may develop in patients with severe hookworm disease. Thick, broad, fused villi, with mucosal atrophy and inflammation of the lamina propria, are seen. If marked chronic anaemia is concurrent, histopathological changes are found in many viscera.

The anaemia of hookworm disease in tropical areas is often profound –and, occasionally, fatal. In patients who are heavily infected with hookworms, blood loss may exceed 200 ml per day, and iron loss may exceed 30 mg daily. The anaemia is closely correlated with the iron loss, since protective haemopoiesis fails only when iron stores are depleted. In the torrid zones this depletion is accelerated by the iron content lost in sweat, by inadequate ferrous absorption due to precipitation in the high phytate and phosphate diets and by losses associated with concomitant parasitic infections. Oral administration of iron will correct the anaemia, but, if therapy is discontinued and the worms are still present, anaemia will recur quickly. On the other hand, the anaemia will persist unchanged if the worms have been eliminated but no iron is administered.

As in any iron deficiency anaemia, the red blood cell morphology is hypochromic and microcytic. The bone marrow reveals normoblastic hyperplasia, with reduction in the myeloid–erythroid ratio and complete absence of free iron. Plasma iron concentration is reduced, while iron-binding capacity is markedly increased. Eosinophilia is often marked but may be decreased or absent when the haemoglobin level has fallen very low.

Combined vermifuge and haematological studies demonstrate a relatively direct correlation between the number of worms infecting the intestine and the amount of blood lost. Since worms are not self-multiplying, as are bacteria, protozoa or viruses, exposure to reinfection is essential for the continuation of the disease. In areas where fields polluted by faeces are common, bare feet the rule and 'night soil' the preferred fertilizer, re-exposure is inevitable. That all natives of the torrid zone are not completely ingested by their worms is due to the development of a poorly understood immunity.

Some clinicians in tropical medicine have been under the impression for many years that an existent hookworm infection provides protection against new infection. Following the same exposure, the white visitor became more heavily infested with worms than did the native. The nature and the extent of acquired immunity to human hookworm infection have not been determined. However, acquired immunity has been clearly demonstrated in animals, and Scottish veterinarians have proved the feasibility of inducing immunity artificially in large-scale vaccination programmes.

Outside tropical areas the question of immunity as a clinical factor is not important. Reinfection is usually impossible, as much because of the sanitary standards as because hookworm eggs do not survive at cool, dry temperatures. Hookworm disease does not persist without reinfection. Diminution in the parasitism will occur after several months in temperate regions and almost always disappear within 2 years. This has obvious therapeutic implications for patients who have taken up permanent residence in temperate climates.

Clinical features

The manifestations of hookworm disease are dermatologic, intestinal and, if anaemia exists, systemic. In an extensive study made in Puerto Rico, the initial skin eruption at the site of larval penetration occurred in 96 per cent of the patients. Vague abdominal pain, anorexia, nausea, flatulence and diarrhoea may occur. If anaemia is present, weakness, lassitude, palpitations, dyspnoea, peripheral and facial oedema and mental and physical retardation are common. In areas where other concomitant parasitic infestations and nutritional deficiencies are the rule, it is impossible to attribute any sign or symptom to hookworm disease alone.

Diagnosis

Laboratory confirmation of hookworm infestation is based on the finding of ova in the stools or adult worms in the faeces after vermifuge. The eggs are oval, with a thin wall, a clear space and a four-celled, granular centre in fresh specimens (Fig. 23). Both *A. duodenale* and *N. americanus* eggs range from 40 to 80 microns in length and cannot be differentiated on direct smear. The eggs are most easily confused with those of *Trichostrongylus* by inexperienced microscopists. The stools should be examined within 24 hours, but, with refrigeration, eggs are identifiable for several weeks. In light infections, concentration techniques of flotation and centrifugation are useful. If only male worms are present, no eggs are found in the stool. If the suspicion of hookworm disease is sufficiently high, and initial stool analyses are negative, a vermifuge may be administered and the faeces examined for adult worms.

The finding of hookworm eggs in a person residing in a nontropical area has little significance unless some estimate of the magnitude of the infestation is given. As was pointed out before, hookworms are not self-multiplying, and the parasite population diminishes rapidly unless there is persistent reinfection. Anthelminthic treatment should not be administered merely because the stool is 'positive for hookworm'. The extent of the infestation and the duration of the infection are essential facts for determining sensible therapy. Stoll has outlined a simple step-by-step egg-counting technique.

Test-tube cultivation is a readily available technique for differentiating between *N. americanus* and *A. duodenale*. Until recently, the de-

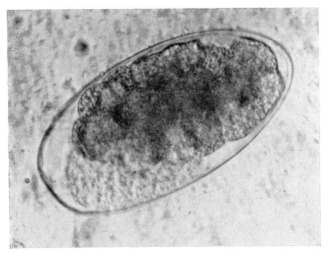

Fig. 23. High-power view of a hookworm egg. The eggs of *Ancylostoma duodenale* and *Necator americanus* are indistinguishable.

termination of which parasite was present was so difficult that no attempt was made before beginning anthelminthic therapy. Now, however, large studies have demonstrated the ease and the value of the test-tube technique of immersing a faeces-stained filter paper in a closed tube, allowing it to incubate and examining the infective larvae as they fall to the bottom. However, the differentiation between larvae is a task for the professional parasitologist only.

Treatment

The determination of which parasite is present is important in selecting proper chemotherapy. Bephenium hydroxynaphthoate (Alcopar) is most effective against *A. duodenale*, whereas tetrachlorethylene is the drug of choice for *N. americanus* infestation. Both drugs should be administered after fasting. The bephenium may be given in a single oral dose of 5 g or, if the patient is under observation, in daily doses for 3 days. The single dose of tetrachlorethylene is 0·1 ml per kg, but it may have to be repeated after 4 days. Purgatives are not necessary. Parasites will be excreted over a period of 4 to 6 days, and the adult worms can be recovered by filtration. Both of the anthelminthics have side-effects of nausea, vomiting, diarrhoea and vertigo. Therefore, it is important to balance the benefits expected from therapy against the side-effects, esepcially in those persons who are not anaemic and are not exposed to reinfection.

Iron-deficiency anaemia from hookworm responds uniformly to 15 to 20 gr of oral ferrous sulphate over a period of 6 to 10 weeks.

BIBLIOGRAPHY

Roche, M., *et al.*   The Nature and Cause of 'Hookworm Anemia'.   *Am. J. trop. Med. Hyg.* **15,** 1209, 1966.
Stoll, N. R.   On Endemic Hookworm: Where Do We Stand Today? *Expl Parasitol.* **12,** 241, 1962.

9   Filariasis

Interest in filarial infections reached a peak toward the end of World War II. Several hundred thousand soldiers had been exposed to the disease, especially in the South Pacific, and 15,000 were known to have had circulating microfilariae. Elaborate plans were devised to cope with the expected hordes developing scrotal and pedal elephantiasis, but these conditions were almost never seen. The only problem that arose was the psychological one of reassuring the frightened soldiers that their sexual life was not impaired.

Awareness of filariasis waned over the next decade, in spite of the fact that the worldwide incidence exceeded 300 million persons. However, as vast populations shifted from endemic filarial zones to temperate climates in the last generation, another 'tropical' infection with chronic manifestations became important in differential diagnosis in America and Europe. In one study in New York City, circulating microfilariae were found in 12 per cent of routine night-blood specimens in asymptomatic Haitian patients.

When there is adequate, successful therapy for the early stages of a disease while, on the other hand, the physical and the psychological deformities of the advanced stages are resistant to treatment, prompt diagnosis and treatment are particularly important. Filariasis is such a disease.

Pathological features

The family Filariidae of the class Nematode includes pathogenic and nonpathogenic parasites of the bloodstream and the tissues of man. *Wuchereria bancrofti*, the major cause of classic filariasis, is transmitted from man to man by the bite of an intermediate host mosquito (*Culex, Aedes* or *Anopheles*). After the mosquito has ingested the blood of an infected man, the parasite develops in the gut and the thoracic muscles of the insect for from 3 to 5 weeks. When the insect then seeks a blood meal, microfilariae migrate along the proboscis and enter the lymphatics of man. Depending on host resistance, the larvae may either die or reach maturity within from 1 to 3 years. At that time, if both male and female adult filariae are present, mating occurs, and swarms of microfilariae can be detected at night. Pathological reactions to the larvae and the adult worms are common, whereas the microfilariae elicit no response.

The earliest evidence of infection is usually noted in the genital and the inguinal lymphatics about 3 months after infection. Transient lymphangitis, often associated with generalized systemic hypersensitivity reactions, occurs with the extension of the inflammation to adjacent vascular channels. Parts of the worm, surrounded by eosinophils and hyperplastic cells, can be identified in lymph node biopsies. As the initial allergic reaction resolves, granulomatous tissue proliferates, causing lymphatic obstruction. Dilatation and variceal formation of dependent lymph channels result. Perilymphangitis, extension phlebitis and phlebothrombosis complicated by secondary bacterial infection are usual. Hyalinization and calcification of the worms eventually occur, causing further fibroblastic proliferation and total obliteration of the involved lymph channels.

Rupture or extravasation from tortuous lymphatics can cause

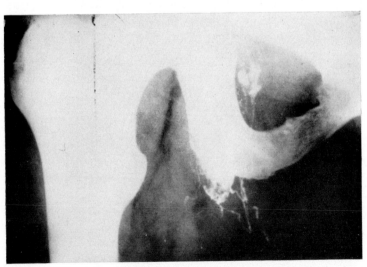

Fig. 24.   Filling defects in an inguinal lymph node, associated with the development of collateral lymph channels, in a patient with filarial elephantiasis of the leg.

oedema of legs and genitalia. The microscopic alterations seen in the skin biopsy of an elephantoid organ or extremity include atrophy of the epidermis, oedema, eosinophilic infiltration of the dermis and, finally, hyperkeratosis and cicatrization over areas of secondary infection resulting in the typical fissured, leatherlike skin.

Lymphangiography with an ultra-fluid oil-soluble dye permits *in vivo* visualization of the lymphatic system of man. In elephantiasis of the leg the main lymphatic channels are replaced by a friable plexus of dermal vessels. Filling defects are found in the inguinal nodes (Fig. 24), apparently related to replacement fibrosis around dead adult worms. In chyluria the para-aortic nodes do not opacify and a diffuse pattern of collateral channels is seen (Fig. 25). The technique of lymphangiography has helped to elucidate the pathogenesis of all phases of the disease.

Clinical features

The clinical manifestations of early filariasis are, at most, nonspecific

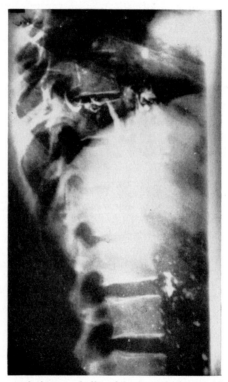

Fig. 25. Abnormal cisterna chyli and horizontal plexus of lymphatics in a patient with filarial chyluria

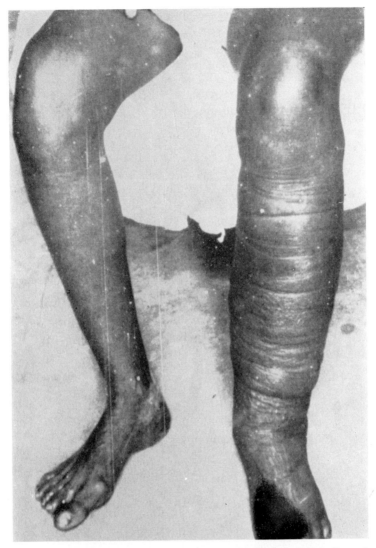

Fig. 26.   Typical elephantoid leg in a patient with filariasis. Thick, fissured and folded leatherlike skin with superficial infection is characteristic.

and, often, nonexistent. There is usually no reaction to the first infection with filarial larvae. However, after sensitization to the initial parasitic invasion, re-exposure to the toxic proteins of the larvae can elicit a systemic allergic reaction. Since so little is known of the pathogenesis of the incubational period, there are few studies of the clinical findings during the first few years of infection. However, it is apparent from the enormous numbers infected and the paucity of complaints that early clinical manifestations are minor.

On the other hand, this is certainly not true of the clinical picture in the acute or the chronic phase. During the acute period of several months there are brief attacks separated by weeks of total remission. Recurrent lymphangitis with visible red streaking, fever, headache,

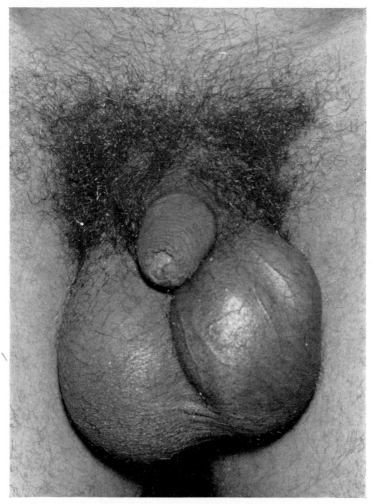

Fig. 27. Scrotal enlargement with visible lymphatic dilatation of the skin and inguinal adenopathy in a patient with filariasis.

myalgias and conjunctivitis are common. The inguinal or the axillary nodes may be palpable and tender. In the male, orchitis, funiculitis and epididymitis are common, and scrotal swelling is frequent. As the duration of the attacks increases, permanent deformities may be observed.

Chronic filariasis is seen only in those patients with repeated attacks of acute lymphangitis and exposure to reinfection for many years in an area where the disease is endemic.

Unilateral pedal elephantiasis and scrotal oedema are the most common end-stages of infection (Figs. 26 and 27). The lesions pictured on these pages are closer to the typical clinical patterns of advanced filariasis than the medical curiosities, such as scrota filling wheelbarrows, often noted in many textbooks. Hydrocele formation is a frequent complication. Chyluria may develop in the presence or the absence of other chronic changes. Because of a lack of awareness of the infection, patients with filariasis are frequently followed as refractory cases in cardiac, urological and renal clinics.

Diagnosis

Unfortunately, the diagnosis of filariasis is often difficult to confirm. This is particularly true in two important groups: those with initial recent exposure to the infection and those with advanced disease. A definitive diagnosis is possible only by demonstrating microfilariae. As was noted earlier, 3 years usually elapse before adult worms are mature and mate. Thus, blood smears in early cases are negative. In the advanced case with complete fibrosis of lymph channels and calcification of adult worms, microfilariae either are not produced or cannot escape into the general circulation.

Microfilariae are present in peripheral blood in large numbers only between 9 p.m. and 2 a.m. The explanations for this nocturnal periodicity are as conjectural today as when Manson first described it in 1878. The theories that are currently propounded are based on the nocturnal biting habits of the *Culex* mosquito, the oxygen saturation of the active versus the resting lung reservoir, and physiological changes in the reproductive cycle of the female *W. bancrofti*. None has been proved. It is interesting to note that the reversal of a man's sleeping and waking schedule will reverse the periodicity of the filarial migration.

The yield of microfilariae can be augmented in borderline cases by increasing the oxygen saturation of the blood and by filtering the blood through fine-pore wire mesh. Blood may be preserved for morning examination by placing 1 ml of blood in 9 ml of a 2 per cent formalin solution. The smears should be made by both thick and thin techniques, and both unstained smears and smears coloured by Giemsa stain should be prepared. If a specimen is examined immediately, the microfilariae may be seen thrashing about without progressive movement. They are cream-white and range from 230 to 290 microns in length (Fig. 28). The anatomical features that differentiate *W. bancrofti* from other filariae are summarized in Table 6, but, since they are

Table 6.   The microfilariae of man

Parasite	Geographic distribution	Site Blood	Site Skin	Sheath	Graceful contour	Tail nucleus
W. bancrofti	Africa, Asia, Americas	x	–	x	x	End < tip
B. malayi	Far East	x	–	x	–	Two terminal nuclei
L. loa	Africa	x	–	x	–	To tip
D. perstans	Africa, Americas	x	–	–	–	End < tip
M. ozzardi	Americas	x	–	–	–	To tip
O. volvulus	Africa, Americas	–	x	–	–	End < tip
D. streptocerca	Africa	–	x	–	–	To tip

complex, a differential diagnosis should be attempted only by an experienced parasitologist.

Ancillary diagnostic methods are dependent on a group-specific immunological response. A wide range of serological tests are available; the bentonite flocculation, indirect haemagglutination and intradermal tests (all employing *Dirofilaria immitis*, a common parasite of the dog, as antigen) are extensively employed. In many cases a clinical picture compatible with filariasis, coupled with a history of exposure in an endemic area, and a positive serological test, must serve as the basis for therapy even if the results of blood smears for microfilariae are negative.

Treatment

Diethylcarbamazine (Hetrazan) is the drug of choice in the treatment of filariasis. Introduced in 1947, it has revolutionized the therapy and the prognosis of the disease. The recommended dosage of 3 mg per kg 3 times daily for 3 weeks will eliminate all circulating microfilariae and have at least an incapacitating, if not lethal, effect on the adult worms. There are no serious toxic reactions to the drug, but mild side-effects such as nausea, vomiting, slight fever, transient urticaria and eosinophilia are common. Treatment should not be discontinued if

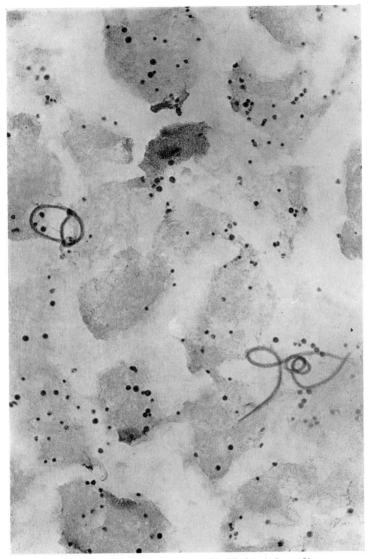

Fig. 28. Thick blood smear with *Wuchereria bancrofti*.

mild side-effects occur. The drug will not affect the elephantiasis of advanced cases.

Supportive measures are essential in therapy of the filarial patient. Elastic stockings, exercise and careful hygiene are necessary measures to prevent breakdown and secondary infection of elephantoid limbs.

75

Plastic surgical treatment of the involved extremities is fraught with the danger of infection, and healing is rarely successful because of the chronic dermal oedema and epidermal atrophy that are present.

Scrotal resection and surgical correction of hydroceles are advisable after chemotherapy has been completed. Recent evidence indicates that the cause of the scrotal oedema is more inflammatory than obstructive

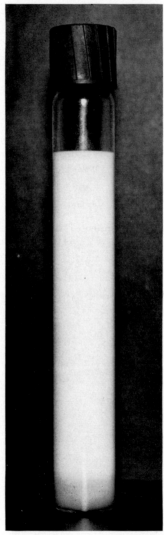

Fig. 29. Chylous urine in filariasis, showing typical layering of blood, chylomicrons and free fat.

in character. Thus, reaccumulation of swelling should not occur if adequate chemotherapy is administered and reinfection does not occur. Reassurance of male patients as to their virility and potential fertility is often of paramount importance. Psychiatric assistance often may be advisable.

There is no uniformly satisfactory treatment for chyluria (Fig. 29). Dietary management with fat intake restricted to medium-chain triglycerides will curtail chyluria in some cases. Although strict bed rest and elevation of the foot of the bed are advised, there is no convincing reason why these practices should be effective, and they have had no appreciable impact on the course of patients with chyluria under our care. Instrumentation will exacerbate an attack, and the surgical stripping of the perinephric lymphatics has no logical basis. One of the great benefits of lymphangiography has been to clarify the site of obstruction and thereby eliminate the extensive and unnecessary surgery formerly advised. Patients with chyluria can lose large amounts of blood as well as significant quantities of fat.

The transient visitor to a filarial region can be reassured that he will develop none of the deformities of chronic wuchereriasis. As noted, not a single case of elephantiasis developed in the 15,000 American soldiers who were known to be infected in World War II, as their exposure to reinfection was less than 3 years. Prophylactic medication against filariasis is not indicated.

Throughout South India and the Malayan peninsula another parasite, *Brugia malayi*, causes elephantiasis. Morphological characteristics differentiating this parasite from *W. bancrofti* are summarized in Table 6. The vectors of *B. malayi* include *Mansonia* mosquitoes as well as *Culex*, *Aedes* and *Anopheles*. The microfilariae do not have a nocturnal periodicity in man. Treatment with diethylcarbamazine is effective.

BIBLIOGRAPHY

Cahill, K., and Kaiser, R.   Lymphangiography in Bancroftian Filariasis.   *Trans. R. Soc. trop. Med. Hyg.* **58,** 356, 1964.
Edeson, J., and Wilson, T.   The Epidemiology of Filariasis due to *W. bancrofti* and *B. malayi*.   *A. Rev. Ent.* **9,** 245, 1964.
Wartman, W. B.   Filariasis in American Armed Forces in World War II.   *Medicine* **26.** 333, 1947.
Jachowski, L. A., Jr, Gonzales-Flores, B., and von Lichtenberg, F.   Filarial Etiology of Tropical Hydroceles in Puerto Rico.   *Am. J. trop. Med.* **11,** 220, 1962.

10 Other Filarial Infections

In addition to wuchereriasis, there are two other filarial infections, onchocerciasis and loiasis, which occur in man in significant numbers. A knowledge of onchocerciasis is essential for any physician dealing with large numbers of Latin Americans; an awareness of both diseases is helpful with patients travelling to and from Africa. Both are chronic diseases, and initial manifestations may appear many years after a person has left a tropical area. Thus, a history of travel and exposure may first arouse the suspicions of the good clinician.

The life cycle of the infecting agents, *Onchocerca volvulus* and *Loa loa*, is similar to that described for *Wuchereria bancrofti*. The major differences are the varying insect vectors and the alteration in microfilarial migration and periodicity. However, the pathological features, the clinical course and the prognosis of the two diseases are quite distinct, and they will be presented separately.

ONCHOCERCIASIS

Only 50 years ago a parasitic disease affecting 75 to 100 per cent of the population in certain communities of Central America was described. Since that time many aspects of the disease have been elucidated. The parasite has been identified and its life cycle determined. The insect vector (various species of *Simulium*, or blackfly) has been found, and its breeding and biting habits have been investigated. Elaborate histological and clinical studies have clarified many features of the pathogenesis of the disease, and several effective drugs for control and treatment have been discovered. Yet the incidence of onchocerciasis today is probably unchanged from the estimates of a half-century ago. It is estimated that 20 million people are affected on the Pacific coasts of Guatemala and Mexico and in Venezuela, the Congo, Liberia, Nigeria, Ghana, the Cameroons, Kenya, Uganda, Tanzania and the Sudan. Because of the ease of travel and the chronic nature of the disease, it is found with increasing frequency in cosmopolitan cities as well as in the areas where it is endemic.

Pathological features. The major pathological changes in onchocerciasis are due either to migration and disintegration of microfilariae or to the death of the adult worm. After a minimal incubation period of 1 year, histological changes may be found in the skin of patients with onchocerciasis. There is thickening of the epidermis, loss of elasticity and, often, fibrous cicatrization caused by an associated pruritic excoriation. Microfilariae lodge in the corium and are surrounded by an eosinophilic infiltration and a generalized perivascular inflammation. Filariae are found with the greatest frequency in the skin of the scapular and lower leg regions, as well as adjacent to subcutaneous nodules.

The formation of nodules is related to the death of the adult worms. Toxins and proteins liberated from a degenerating *O. volvulus* in the subcutaneous tissue elicit an inflammatory response. Histological sections reveal leukocytic infiltration, fibroblastic proliferation and eventual granulomatous formation. In chronic nodules there may be caseation and calcification. The majority of nodules in African onchocerciasis are on the trunk and the legs, while almost all in Central America are found on the head and the scalp. The reason for this distribution is unknown. It has been claimed that there is an association between the incidence of scalp nodules and blindness.

Pathological changes in the eyes have been associated with onchocerciasis since the discovery of the disease. For many years it was considered to be a late but almost inevitable complication of chronic infection. Recent evidence has indicated that ocular involvement may also be an initial symptom and that it may be found in light infections. In the anterior segment, punctate keratitis, corneal opacification, iritis, sclerosing limbitis and glaucoma may occur. There is no involvement of the lens. In the posterior segment, chorioretinitis and optic atrophy have been widely attributed to *O. volvulus* infection, although the pathogenesis of these lesions has not yet been fully explained. The prevalence of syphilis, trachoma and nutritional deficiencies may account for some of the blindness in communities where onchocerciasis is a concomitant disease. However, epidemiological evidence strongly supports the contention that onchocerciasis is the cause of the 'river blindness' which comes from optic atrophy and is found in up to 10 per cent of the village populations in areas where onchocerciasis is endemic.

Clinical features. Onchocercal keratitis and the very minute opacifications from dead microfilariae are rarely associated with any change in visual acuity. The gradual development of blindness is a feature of heavy infection and pathological changes in the posterior segment. Onchocercal keratitis is usually painless, but photophobia, conjunctivitis and epiphora may occur.

Pruritus is the most common symptom (in 70 per cent), with the back and the thighs most frequently involved. These are the areas, it will be

79

recalled, where microfilariae are most easily demonstrable. A rash may or may not coexist; the same is true for subcutaneous nodules. Since nodules were the diagnostic feature in early reports, it was long held that they were found in 100 per cent of these patients. However, in a recent survey, nodules were noted in only 23 per cent, and their presence is certainly not essential in making a diagnosis of onchocerciasis. In fact, they may appear only after adequate therapy has caused the death of the adult worm.

Diagnosis. Demonstration of the microfilariae of *O. volvulus* on skin biopsy confirms the diagnosis of onchocerciasis. A thin section of skin (so superficial as not to cause bleeding) should be excised from the scapular area, the upper thighs or over nodules and should be mounted in saline and examined directly with the microscope. Alternative methods include examination of the lymph from a scarified site, the making of histological sections through a nodule (Fig. 30) or visualization of filariae or onchocercal keratitis when there is ocular involvement. Serological tests (with *Dirofilaria immitis* as antigen) are useful as a screening measure. A negative test result provides strong evidence against infection, while a positive test result indicates a more intensive search for the parasite. Cross-reactions with other filarial infections have already been commented upon, and interpretation of results depends upon clinical and epidemiological facts in each case. An eosinophilia of over 10 per cent is usually present in active infection.

Treatment. Diethylcarbamazine (Hetrazan) is the drug of choice for onchocerciasis. As with wuchereriasis, its action is primarily on the microfilaria, with death of the adult worm occurring, rarely, after one course of therapy—more usually after several. Allergic reactions are the rule rather than the exception and may be serious when there are ocular lesions. When the eyes are not involved, the initial dosage should be 1 mg per kg of body weight, and this should be increased rapidly to a daily dose of 10 mg per kg by the fourth day. This should be continued for 2 weeks, and a second course should be given after an interval of 2 weeks. When the eyes are involved, the initial dose should be smaller and the increments should be made more slowly. Allergic manifestations are usually controllable with antihistamines, but cortisone may be necessary to diminish severe ocular reactions.

After microfilarial elimination, the adult worm can be destroyed by intravenous administration of Antrypol. The usual effective regimen is a weekly injection of 1 g (10 per cent solution) for 5 weeks. The drug has definite renal toxicity, and pre-existing kidney disease is a contraindication. The urine should be checked to ensure that it is free of

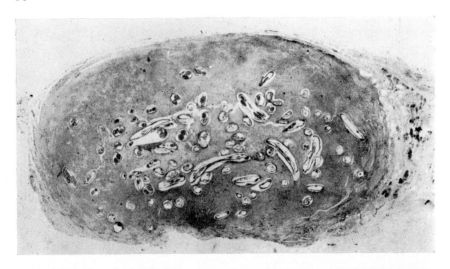

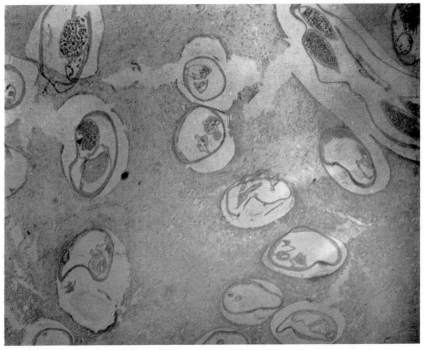

Fig. 30.   *Top,* cross-section of an onchocercal nodule; *bottom,* detail of nodule, showing segments of adult *Onchocerca volvulus* worms.

protein before each injection. If either drug is administered alone, there is a high incidence of relapse. However, with combination therapy and without reinfection, the cure rate exceeds 90 per cent. Since the nodule arises from degenerating worms, surgical extirpation does not remove a source of continuing parasitic production.

There is no effective drug prophylaxis for patients visiting rural areas where the disease is endemic. The sole practical preventive measure is to avoid being bitten by the *Simulium* fly. Insect repellents for skin and clothes such as diethyltoluamide are effective for less than 12 hours and must be reapplied frequently. Insecticide spraying of sleeping quarters is of no use, and mosquito nets over beds should be advised. Adequate clothing should be worn on hiking trips, to cover exposed skin.

LOIASIS

In many of the wet, wooded areas of Africa, another filarial infection, loiasis, is found. Transmitted by the day-biting female deerfly, *Chrysops*, the microfilariae *L. loa* have a diurnal periodicity in man. The life cycle of the parasite is similar to that described for *W. bancrofti* except that the larvae lodge in connective and muscular tissues rather than in the lymphatics during the one year required for maturation.

Pathological and clinical features. Migrations of the adult worm are responsible for the occasional pathological features of loiasis. In the majority of infected patients the parasite wanders in the soft tissues of the body without eliciting either a histological or a clinical response. Transient erythema and pruritus may occur in the skin above the worm; oedema, conjunctivitis and pain accompany the ocular migrations of the parasite. *L. loa* have been found in almost all tissues of the body, and a wide variety of unusual signs and symptoms have been reported from areas where loiasis is endemic. The most consistent manifestation of the disease is the development of subcutaneous nodules (Calabar swellings), usually appearing after exercise or on exposure to heat and disappearing within 3 days; they may or may not be painful. The pathogenesis of these lesions is most probably of an allergic nature similar to that described for onchocercal nodules. However, live *L. loa* can be found in many Calabar swellings, so that the antigen–antibody reaction in these nodules is not always due to degenerating parasites as in onchocerciasis. Calabar swellings may be induced in a patient with loiasis by a subcutaneous injection of *D. immitis* solution.

Diagnosis. Once again, demonstration of the parasite is the only

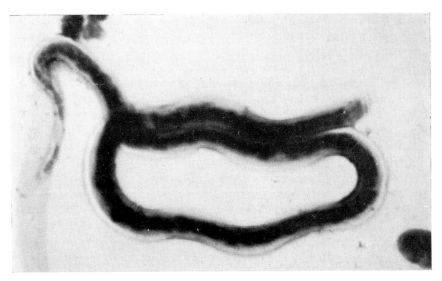

Fig. 31A   Oil-immersion view of *Loa loa* in the blood of a West African patient.

definitive method of diagnosis. Visible adult worms may be removed from ocular or cutaneous sites, and microfilariae may be found on thick, diurnal, peripheral blood smears or on scrapings from Calabar swellings (Fig. 31A). The yield of microfilariae can be increased by straining the blood through a fine mesh filter which retains the parasite. An eosinophilia of over 20 per cent is invariably present in infected patients. Serological tests have the same advantages and disadvantages as have been noted for other filarial infections.

Treatment. Diethylcarbamazine is highly effective in loiasis, causing the death of both microfilariae and adult worms. Allergic reactions to the degenerating parasites are so common that antihistamines should be administered for the first 4 days of the 10-day regimen. Patients visiting regions where loiasis is endemic should be aware of the biting habits of *Chrysops* in order to avoid infection. Since the deerflies do not travel far from the forest edge, a 200-yard clearing around the camp provides excellent protection. The fly bites only during the day, so that adequate clothing and insect repellent are essential during this period.

RELATED INFESTATIONS

Rare cases of human infection with the canine parasites, *Dirofilaria immitis* and *D. conjunctivae*, have been reported. In the few cases detected

in the southern United States, the diagnosis was made from morphological characteristics of worms removed from the conjunctiva and the
subcutaneous tissues.

The oldest known filarial infection of man is dracontiasis, or guinea
worm disease. The parasite *Dracunculus medinensis* infects man over a
wide area of Africa, India, and Latin America and has been found in
several species of wild animals in the United States. Over 50 million
people are estimated to be afflicted with the guinea worm. Infection
follows the ingestion of water contaminated with infected *Cyclops*, the
liberation of the parasite in the intestine, and its migration to and
maturation in subcutaneous tissues. The adult worm bores to the
surface of an extremity and eventually erupts through a pruritic blister.

Traditional treatment has been limited to aiding the evacuation by
coiling the worm around a solid instrument and pulling (Fig. 31B).
However, failure to remove the entire parasite is common, and secondary infection is then the rule. Various modifications, including prior
freezing of the skin with ethyl chloride, superficial dissection and

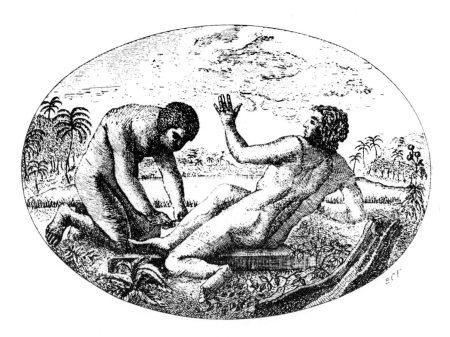

Fig. 31B   *Extraction of the Guinea Worm* (from an engraving by J. H. Jördens,
1802). The current therapy for dracontiasis is unchanged from this primitive
worm-extraction technique.

rhythmic dermal massage, enhance the expulsion of the entire worm. Diethylcarbamazine has been used but has not been consistently effective. Thiabendazole (Mintezol) has been successfully employed in several large series with a total dose of 3 g in a 25 mg/kg twice-daily regimen. Visitors to areas where the disease is endemic should be advised to boil their drinking water.

Tropical pulmonary eosinophilia (T.P.E.) is a clinical diagnosis; a single specific aetiological agent fulfilling Koch's postulates has not been identified. However, most evidence incriminates a variety of nonhuman filarial parasites eliciting a hypersensitivity reaction in an aberrant site and host. The clinical syndrome of T.P.E. consists of a paroxysmal cough often associated with dyspnoea and bronchial constriction, fever, perspiration and malaise. Rhonchi and evidence of apical effusion may be elicited. Chest X-ray reveals a characteristic miliary mottling in about half the cases. The white blood cell count usually exceeds 30,000 with a prominent eosinophilia. The filarial complement-fixation test is positive; diethylcarbamazine is curative, and this provides even further supportive evidence for the filarial aetiology of T.P.E.

BIBLIOGRAPHY

Nelson, G. S.   Onchocerciasis.   *Adv. Parasitol.* **8,** 173, 1970.
Choyce, D.   Onchocerciasis.   *Trans. ophthalm. Soc., U.K.* **84,** 371, 1964.
Raffier, G.   Thiabendazole in Dracunculiasis.   *Tex. Rep. Biol. Med.* **27,** 601, 1969.

11   Other Nematode Infections

Most of mankind harbour at least one helminth. Some of these parasites are responsible for significant morbidity and mortality throughout the world; important examples of this group of diseases, including schistosomiasis, hookworm disease, filariasis and echinococcosis, have been considered separately.

In addition to hookworm and filarial parasites, which have been considered previously, man can serve as both a natural and an accidental host to other nematodes. Human disease may follow the ingestion of infective eggs or contaminated meat, invasion by infective larvae and, occasionally, autoinfection and retroinfection. The identification of adult nematodes is an easy task for the tropical disease expert, and essential details of size and oesophageal and buccal contours are available in any textbook of parasitology. They will not be repeated here, since the physician and the casual student of tropical medicine are unlikely to see the adult worms and will diagnose infections by clinical patterns and egg morphology. In the following sections, the diseases are presented in the order of decreasing frequency and importance to the temperate-climate clinician.

ENTEROBIASIS

Pinworm is a common parasite, with a particularly high incidence of infection in closed communities such as boarding schools and mental hospitals. Enterobiasis is more prevalent in the temperate zone than in the tropics and, for some as yet unexplained reason, is found more frequently in white persons than in Negroes or Latin Americans living under identical conditions. Man is the only host of *Enterobius vermicularis*. Infection is transmitted from man to man by the anal–oral route. This may be accomplished by handling contaminated sheets or pyjamas or inhaling egg-laden dust, as well as by a direct hand-to-mouth method. Migration of larvae back through the anus accounts for rare retroinfection.

An ingested egg hatches in the duodenum, and the worm matures in the caecum. As the female worm becomes gravid, it migrates through the anus to deposit its eggs on the perianal skin. The adult worm crawls actively among its discharge for several hours before dying. This movement elicits a severe pruritic reaction, and, as the patient scratches, the fingernails become contaminated with eggs, thereby allowing an easy route for the life cycle of reinfection to begin again.

Diagnosis and treatment. The adult worm produces only minimal pathological changes in the caecum, and excoriation with secondary infection is an unusual perianal complication; however, a wide range of generalized symptoms—mostly psychological—have been attributed to pinworm infection. Diagnosis is made by visualizing eggs in stool examinations, on rectal swabs or on transparent tape preparations (Fig. 32). The last-mentioned procedure should be performed immediately on arising in the morning. A simple method is the application of a small piece of Scotch tape to the perianal area; then the tape is

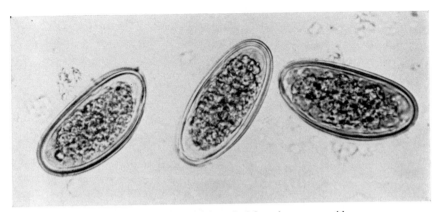

Fig. 32. Pinworm ova with typical flat edges on one side.

fixed to a glass slide before microscopy. Individual infections can be cured by a course of piperazine citrate (Antepar) in a daily dose of 65 mg per kg for 7 days. The liquid adipate compound is often desirable for children. An alternative effective drug, pyrvinium pamoate (Povan), is also available. Both mass treatment and a rigorous daily programme of scrupulous personal hygiene must be instituted. Nails must be clipped close and clothing and towels carefully segregated and changed daily. Since pinworm eggs have thick, chitinous shells, they are quite resistant to time and temperature, and will survive in the cracks of floors or in rugs even after casual cleaning. I advise patients to follow a thorough cleansing, particularly of the bathroom and bedroom, which are most likely to be contaminated, with heat. An electric heater elevating the room temperature to 90°F will crack the egg walls. These measures are imperative in closed communities if rapid reinfection is to be avoided.

ASCARIASIS

Ascaris lumbricoides is the roundworm most commonly found in man. It is conservatively estimated that over 600 million persons are infected; of this number some 3 million are indigenous cases in the United States, and a larger group, having acquired the parasite abroad, immigrate or return there from vacations in the less sanitary tropics. In wide areas of Asia, Africa and Latin America almost 100 per cent of the population have ascariasis. Fortunately, the parasite produces few clinical

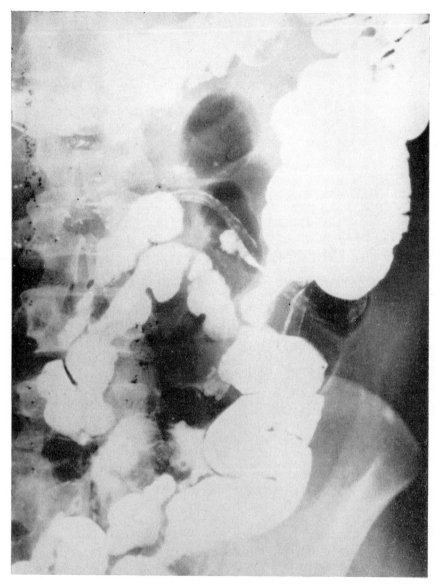

Fig. 33. An adult ascaris outlined in the small intestine by a barium X-ray study.

symptoms, except during the initial invasive phase or when infection is so heavy that mechanical obstruction or aberrant localization occurs.

Man is infected by swallowing an infective *A. lumbricoides* egg. This hatches in the duodenum and the resultant rhabditiform larva penetrates the gut wall, enters the portal circulation, and, having passed through the liver and the heart, reaches the lung in from 7 to 8 days. Here it penetrates an alveolus, enters the bronchial tree, migrates or is coughed up the trachea, and is swallowed. Back in the intestine the adults mature and mate, and each gravid female is producing 200,000 eggs per day within 6 to 8 weeks of infection. The eggs must mature in soil for 4 to 5 weeks before they become infective to man; they can remain viable for from 7 to 10 years.

During the migratory phase the larvae may elicit a hypersensitivity reaction, with urticaria, asthma and eosinophilia. Occasionally, penetration of the alveolar wall is associated with haemoptysis and may be complicated by bacterial infection, the so-called ascaris pneumonia. Heavy infestation with adult worms can cause a variety of gastro-intestinal disturbances including nausea, vomiting, diarrhoea or constipation, colic and, when a mass of worms is large enough to block the small bowel, signs and symptoms of acute intestinal obstruction (Fig. 33). Worms may migrate up the biliary tree, causing a chronic cholecystitis and, occasionally, hepatic abscess; they may block the lumen of the appendix; in malnourished infants they have been incriminated as a cause of intestinal perforation. One of the most effective means of provoking adult ascaris movement is anaesthesia and manipulation of the bowel at surgery. Stool examination and treatment (if indicated) should precede any operative procedure on a patient who comes from or has visited the tropics.

Diagnosis is made by observing ova in stool smears (Fig. 34).

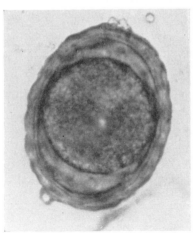

Fig. 34.   Egg of *Ascaris lumbricoides*.

Treatment with piperazine is highly effective; the regimen outlined for pinworm is advised.

TRICHINOSIS

Trichinosis is the only parasitic disease that is more common in the United States than anywhere else in the world. Also peculiar to trichinosis among nematode infections is the fact that man is both the intermediate and the definitive host of the parasite. Man acquires trichinosis by eating inadequately cooked pork, or more rarely bear meat, containing the larval cysts of *Trichinella spiralis*. One of the most common sources of infection is the tasting of home-made sausage during its preparation; the disease has been particularly common among German housewives. The larvae exist in the duodenum, burrow into the intestinal mucosa, mature and mate; and, within a few weeks, a gravid female is producing new larvae. These travel via the blood and the lymphatic systems to the liver, the lungs, the striated musculature and the central nervous system (Fig. 35).

The adult worms rarely produce signs and symptoms; transient diarrhoea and vague abdominal discomfort may initiate heavy infections. However, the migration of larvae is marked by fever, myalgia,

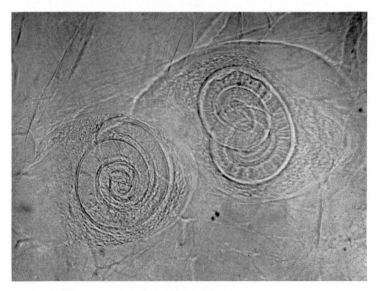

Fig. 35.   Trichinella larvae in a fresh-pressed preparation of muscle.

orbital oedema, conjunctivitis, photophobia, signs of pneumonitis and pleuritis, diarrhoea and, occasionally, evidence of myocarditis. Patients with heavy infections may die during this period from cardiac arrhythmia and congestive heart failure. Muscular aches and pains may persist during the 6-month encystment stage.

Diagnosis may be made by muscle biopsy, complement-fixation, precipitation, flocculation and skin tests. Thiabendazole (Mintezol) is an effective oral anthelminthic that destroys larvae of *Trichinella*. Since the severity of clinical trichinosis varies so widely, depending upon the intensity of infection and the stage of disease when the patient consults the physician, it is difficult to be dogmatic regarding recommended dosage. One might begin at 25 mg/kg, and continue for up to 5 days. Nausea, vomiting and skin rashes are common side-effects of therapy, and the death of multiple larvae releases foreign protein that can result in severe anaphylactic reactions. These must often be controlled with cortisone and antihistamines.

STRONGYLOIDIASIS

The diagnosis of strongyloidiasis is difficult. Patients with the disease are only rarely symptomatic and then in a nonspecific fashion; furthermore, the parasite does not produce an easily identifiable egg in faeces but, rather, an elusive larva which is detected in at least 20 per cent of cases only by duodenal drainage.

Strongyloides stercoralis worms live in the upper small intestine; only the female parasite has been described in man. Human infection most frequently follows the penetration of bare feet by infective larvae. The parasite is then carried through the liver–heart–lung–intestine route outlined for *A. lumbricoides*. Mature worms presumably mate in the duodenum (though the male has not been isolated) and produce rhabditiform larvae. Alternative methods of larval invasion include (a) autoinfection through the bowel or the perianal skin and (b) penetration of the skin by infective larvae produced by male and female adult parasites in a free-living cycle in the soil.

Larvae may elicit an allergic reaction at the site of penetration and also during the migratory phase. The most common manifestations are localized urticarial wheal, eosinophilia and, rarely, pneumonitis. Adult worms may produce a spastic duodenitis with nausea, vomiting, epigastric pain, diarrhoea or constipation. Severe gastrointestinal symptoms including dysentery, ileus and rectal prolapse may occur in undernourished children with massive infections. Occasional 'over-whelming' strongyloidiasis develops with hepatic and pulmonary involvement. Irregular exacerbations follow autoinfections.

Diagnosis is made by finding larvae in fresh faecal specimens. It is important to examine fresh material, since hookworm larvae can emerge from their eggs within hours of defecation; although morphological details permit the differentiation of hookworm and strongyloid larvae, this requires an experienced parasitologist. However, even the casual observer can be assured of a diagnosis of strongyloidiasis if larvae are found in freshly passed stool.

Oral treatment with thiabendazole is highly effective. For intestinal infections 25 mg/kg twice daily for 3 days is recommended. For overwhelming infections a longer course is necessary.

TRICHIASIS

The whipworm of man, *Trichuris trichiura*, is a common intestinal nematode with an infection rate in many Asiatic areas exceeding 50 per cent of the population. Fortunately, the disease is symptomatic only when parasitism is heavy.

Man is the major host of *T. trichiura*, and infection is transmitted from man to man via the anal–oral route. Eggs passed in the stool must

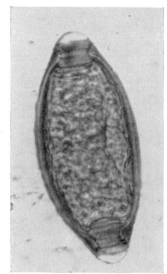

Fig. 36.   Whipworm ovum with typical 'plugs' at both ends.

mature in moist soil for from 2 to 4 weeks before infective larvae develop. When embryonate eggs are ingested, the larvae escape in the duodenum; as the parasite develops, it migrates to the caecal area. Here the adult worm may live for several years, sucking nourishment through a whip-like anterior portion from the host's intestinal mucosa.

The caecum becomes hyperaemic; in heavy infections the mucosa may erode, slough and bleed; in massive infections the entire colon is affected and rectal prolapse is common. Eosinophilia is in proportion to the intensity of infection. Nonspecific abdominal pain, diarrhoea and, occasionally, dysentery occur.

Diagnosis is made by visualization of a whipworm egg on faecal examination (Fig. 36). Eggs are usually plentiful, and the double-plugged lemon shape is easily distinguished from other ova. Treatment with thiabendazole, as outlined for strongyloidiasis, is suggested.

LARVA MIGRANS

Nematodes of dogs and cats occasionally parasitize man. Since man is an unnatural host for these roundworms, the parasites localize in aberrant sites and elicit a strong allergic response. Dependent on the mode of infection, two distinct syndromes, cutaneous larva migrans and visceral larva migrans, result.

Cutaneous larva migrans, or creeping eruption, is due to the movement of canine or feline hookworm larvae in the skin of man. In the southern United States and the Caribbean *Ancylostoma braziliensis* is the common causative parasite; *Uncinaria stenocephala* (the European dog worm), *A. caninum* and *Gnathostoma spinigerum* may also be responsible. Human infection is often associated with exposure of sunbathers, children or workers to contaminated beaches, sandboxes or soil, respectively. The larvae enter the epidermis but are unable to penetrate the stratum germanitivum. They migrate in the epidermis for several days, causing elevated, pruritic, serpiginous channels along the skin surface. An intense eosinophilic reaction occurs.

Treatment aims at effective control of allergic symptoms and killing of the parasite. Antihistamines will accomplish the former aim; thiabendazole is the drug of choice for the latter. Local freezing of the lesion with ethyl chloride and systemic treatment with tetrachlorethy-lene, chloroquine and diethylcarbamazine have been less successfully employed.

Visceral larva migrans results from the ingestion of embryonate

93

eggs of canine or feline ascarids. Children who have been playing in and eating dirt account for the majority of patients with visceral larva migrans. The parasite which is incriminated most frequently is *Toxocara canis*.

The eggs hatch in the duodenum and the larvae penetrate the gut wall, beginning the ascarid cycle of development. However, since man is an unnatural host, larvae are blocked in lungs, liver or aberrant sites, such as the eye, by an intense eosinophilic, granulomatous reaction. The clinical picture is one of low-grade, persistent fever with hepatomegaly, cough and a high eosinophilia. Unilateral ocular enlargement, which is often confused with an orbital tumour, can occur.

Diagnosis is based on histological identification of *T. canis* in biopsy material and is supported by positive serological reactions to ascaris or toxocara antigens. Therapy with thiabendazole is effective.

BIBLIOGRAPHY

Marsden, P.   Intestinal Parasites.   *Gastroenterology* **57,** 724, 1969.
Symons, L.   Pathology of Gastrointestinal Helminthiases.   *Int. Rev. trop. Med.* **3,** 49, 1969.
Gould, S. E.   *Trichinosis in Man and Animals*.   Springfield, Ill., Charles C. Thomas, 1970.
Cahill, K.   Thiabendazole in Strongyloidiasis.   *Am. J. trop. Med. Hyg.* **16,** 451, 1967.
Jackson, G., *et al. Immunity to Parasitic Animals*.   2 vol., New York, Appleton-Century-Crofts, 1969, 1970.

12   Manson's Schistosomiasis

In many parts of South America, and the Caribbean, throughout Africa and the Middle East, and in vast areas of Asia, schistosomal infections are a clinical and economic curse. Over a million persons throughout the world are infected, and the global incidence, in contrast with other parasitic disease, is rising. It is likely to increase even more in the foreseeable future as irrigation and reclamation projects in the developing lands allow wider dissemination of suitable snail vectors, and as inexpensive mass transportation permits the worldwide dissemination of infected human hosts.

The clinical challenge of schistosomiasis in temperate climates is epitomized by the experience of New York City, where over one million migrants from Puerto Rico, a highly endemic schistosomiasis area, have settled in the past two decades. The relatively long incubation period of the disease, combined with the speed and availability of international travel, makes a knowledge of the acute manifestations of schistosomiasis essential for the good clinician. Since active disease may exist for 30 years after the initial infection, with pathological changes in many organs of the body, the detection rate of chronic schistosomiasis among exposed groups should be in direct proportion to an awareness of the possibility.

Recent improvements in laboratory methods of diagnosis and advances in pharmacological and surgical therapy contribute to the current challenge of schistosomiasis. Finally, physicians in Europe and America have an unusual opportunity to study the natural history of the disease in a large population harbouring the parasite but no longer exposed to reinfection.

Three species of *Schistosoma*, *S. mansoni*, *S. haematobium* and *S. japonicum*, cause significant disease in man. Manson's schistosomiasis will be considered first.

Pathological features

A freshwater snail is a necessary intermediate vector in the transmission of schistosomiasis. Appropriate snails for *S. mansoni* are found only in Africa, Arabia, northeastern South America, the West Indies and Puerto Rico. The life cycle of the parasite commences when the schistosomal eggs, passed in excreta by the infected human definitive host into a body of fresh water, hatch miracidia. The miracidia enter the intermediate host snail and, in approximately 1 month, liberate numerous motile, infective cercariae. In this stage of development the parasite can enter another human, either by penetrating the skin of a person who is wading or in contaminated drinking water. Within 3 weeks the cercariae mature into adult worms, and, after copulation, eggs are produced and passed into the faeces of the human being, thus completing the life cycle.

The pathophysiological manifestations of schistosomiasis last from the moment of entry of the cercariae until long after the evacuation of the final egg. As the head of the cercaria penetrates the human skin (its body and tail disengage), an acute inflammatory reaction occurs. An urticarial wheal may develop, with marked leukocytic infiltration in the stratum corneum and the basal layer of the epidermis. The larvae are swept through lymphatic and vascular channels to the liver, where they mature for 2 to 3 weeks. Histological changes during this phase of

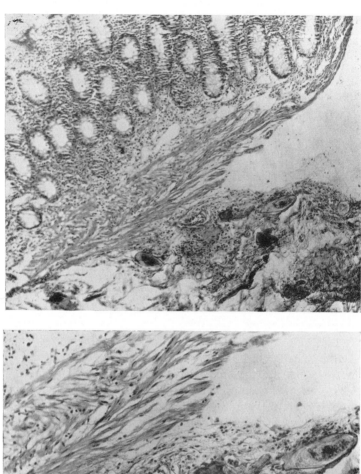

Fig. 37. Rectal mucosal biopsy showing, *top*, ulceration and inflammation and, *bottom*, invasion by lateral-spined schistosoma.

development are caused by the local migratory movements of the parasite and by general sensitization reactions. Small areas of haemorrhage and localized inflammation with acute visceral distention may be found in the liver, the lungs and the spleen. Peripheral eosinophilia, urticaria and bronchial constriction form part of the picture of widespread allergic disease.

The adult worms migrate from the liver against the portal stream to their final resting-place in the inferior haemorrhoidal and mesenteric vessels. There is little reaction to the intravascular adult worms. However, as the female parasite produces eggs, acute and chronic changes occur. The exact mechanism of intestinal penetration by ova that were deposited in the mesenteric vessels is unknown. A lytic substance secreted by the egg elicits an inflammatory reaction, with neutrophilic and eosinophilic infiltration, formation of submucosal abscesses, oedema, hypertrophy and petechial haemorrhage of the mucosa (Fig. 37). Eggs which have been swept back into the circulatory system produce foci of hepatic necrosis around the portal veins and incite pseudo-tubercle formation. This characteristic lesion consists of the necrotic egg surrounded by epithelioid and giant cells, with connective tissue proliferation. At least part of the hepatic and much of the systemic reaction during this acute phase of schistosomiasis is an immunological reaction of the delayed hypersensitivity type. Eosinophilia, urticaria, pyrexia, and vascular and bronchiolar constriction are frequently noted.

The cumulative damage from multiple acute episodes of egg deposition in the bowel produces the pathological manifestations of chronic intestinal schistosomiasis. The colonic wall becomes thickened, rigid and fibrotic, and the mucosa is often granular and friable. Polyps, bowel strictures and rectal prolapse are occasional complications.

The severity of chronic schistosomal liver damage bears only a slight relationship to the extent of parasitic infection. Proliferation and cicatrization around pseudotubercles result in periportal fibrosis, clay-pipe-stem cirrhosis and portal hypertension. Schistosomal liver disease is almost unique in the extent of portal hypertension, presinusoidal block of the blood flow, and granuloma reaction (Fig. 38), but with large areas of perfectly normal liver parenchyma and characteristically normal liver function tests. In tropical disease areas where malnutrition and multiple parasitic infections are the rule, it is extremely difficult to ascribe diffuse pathological alterations to one cause. Controlled animal experiments and studies in man outside endemic areas indicate that by far the major hepatic damage is caused by the schistosome egg, and the

97

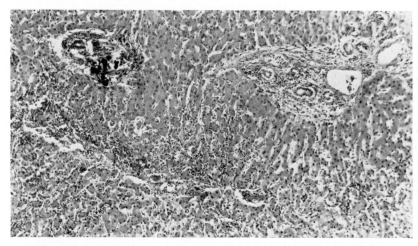

Fig. 38. Hepatic schistosomiasis with interlobular fibrosis, vascular dilatation and calcified ova.

accompanying immunological response and secondary ischaemia. As cirrhosis develops and portal hypertension rises, hypersplenism may occur, and gastric, oesophageal and haemorrhoidal varices form as collateral blood channels. Rupture of oesophageal and gastric varices accentuates the hepatic ischaemia in chronic schistosomiasis.

Dilatation of the haemorrhoidal plexus and evolution of porto-pulmonary anastomoses in the patient with cirrhosis provide direct channels for parasitic dissemination to the lungs. The ova incite an allergic arteriolitis and, eventually, an obliterative granulomatous arteritis, again an immunological reaction of the delayed hyper-sensitivity type (Fig. 39). Pulmonary hypertension and secondary right ventricular enlargement (cor pulmonale) develop.

Schistosomal granulomas occasionally involve the nervous system, usually in the form of expanding spinal cord tumours. Bizarre *S. mansoni* lesions of the brain, the genitalia, the skin and the viscera are sufficiently rare to deserve report in the literature.

Clinical features

The most common clinical finding in Manson's schistosomiasis occurs with the initial infection. Over 95 per cent of Puerto Rican patients in one study had a pruritic dermatitis at the time of cercarial penetration. A transient macular eruption is frequent, and, occasionally, diffuse erythema and urticaria occur. Since this reaction lasts less than

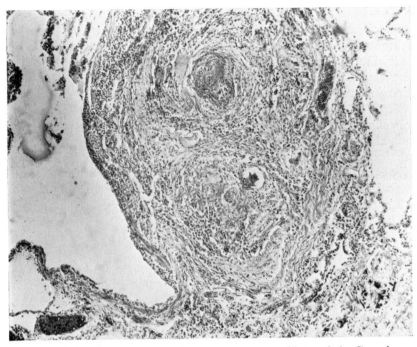

Fig. 39. Pseudotubercle formation in pulmonary schistosomiasis. Central calcified ovum, peripheral leukocytic infiltration and granulomatous change are characteristic.

24 hours, it is rarely seen except in regions where the disease is endemic. Later manifestations of the disease are neither specific nor consistent.

Depending on the degree of host resistance, signs and symptoms may or may not occur during the phase of parasitic migration, maturation and egg deposition. A severe reaction may include fever, abdominal pain, cough, haemoptysis, urticarial rash, headache, malaise, anorexia, recurrent diarrhoea with faecal blood and mucus, tenesmus and hepatosplenomegaly. Evidence of chronic infection is also diffuse and, in those with severe intestinal and hepatic lesions, includes haematemesis, melaena, ascites, weight loss, malaise, alternating diarrhoea and constipation, pallor and fever. Pulmonary involvement may result in failure of the right side of the heart, with dyspnoea and syncope on exertion, haemoptysis and cyanosis. In the rare patient with involvement of the central nervous system or other unusual sites, clinical findings are appropriate to the pathological changes.

Diagnosis

Visualization of eggs is necessary for the diagnosis of Manson's schistosomiasis. Haematological and immunological tests may provide the initial evidence of infection and the stimulus for an intensive search for the parasite. Nevertheless, the morphological identification of *S. mansoni* remains the only certain basis for diagnosis.

Six to 8 weeks after primary infection, lateral-spined ova of *S. mansoni* may be detectable in the stool. Since it is not primarily a luminal parasite, eggs may be few in number, and concentrating techniques increase the positive yield. The easiest method is a double sedimentation in lukewarm tap water, with straining through standard surgical gauze. When the supernatant clears (in approximately 30 to 40 minutes) the sediment is examined under the microscope. Since eggs will hatch into miracidia within 4 hours, microscopy should not be delayed. The ova are yellow-brown and elongated (100 × 60 microns) and have a prominent lateral spine (Fig. 40).

Alternative methods of detecting ova in the rectal mucosa include microscopy of mucus removed by digital or instrument manipulation

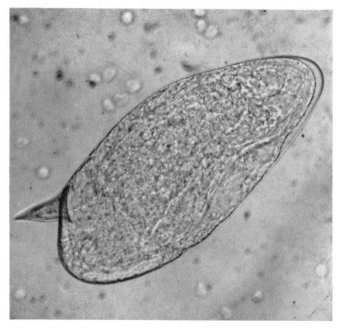

Fig. 40. High-power view of *Schistosoma mansoni* egg demonstrating typical lateral spine.

and direct examination of a proctoscopic snip of a rectal valve pressed between 2 slides. Half of the rectal biopsy specimen should be examined directly and the remainder preserved for histological sections (Fig. 37). Inspection with the sigmoidoscope may reveal a characteristic granular mucosa, with small punctate haemorrhages and isolated ulcerations. Polyps are uncommon, and sigmoidoscopic findings will be normal in at least 50 per cent of patients with chronic schistosomiasis. Percutaneous liver biopsy is a useful and safe method of assessing hepatic involvement in advanced schistosomiasis (Fig. 38) but should not serve as a substitute for faecal or rectal examination.

Immunological tests using cercariae and adult worms as antigenic substance are of many varieties: intradermal and serological methods including direct and indirect haemagglutination, circumoval precipitin, complement-fixation, bentonite flocculation, and fluorescent antibody tests have all been widely used and have demonstrated in epidemiological surveys a specificity and sensitivity of 90 per cent or better. The WHO has released a standardized antigen (Melcher's acid-soluble protein fraction) for serological testing. False positive and false negative test results can occur, and, in view of the toxicity of available therapy, a decision on therapy should not be based solely on these tests. However, a positive serological result in a patient in whom stool and biopsy examinations show a negative result demands vigorous reinvestigation and repetition of standard diagnostic measures.

Blood tests provide ancillary evidence of infection in both the early and the late phases of schistosomiasis. Eosinophilia during the acute stage of maturation and egg deposition usually exceeds 15 per cent but may be normal in the patient with chronic disease. Anaemia from schistosomiasis alone is rare. The sedimentation rate is usually elevated, and an increased gamma globulin fraction on protein electrophoresis is characteristic. Liver function tests in the patient with hepatic schistosomiasis are usually normal.

Splenic photography can outline the vascular complications of schistosomal cirrhosis. The investigation of the more usual sites of *S. mansoni* infection may require a wide variety of appropriate tests.

Treatment

The diagnosis of Manson's schistosomiasis is not always an indication for therapy. In Puerto Rico, for example, most infected patients are completely asymptomatic, and, in view of the toxicity of available chemotherapy, drug treatment is recommended only in advanced disease with splenomegaly. Certainly, in non-endemic areas where the patient is no longer exposed to the cumulative insults of reinfection, the treatment may well be worse than the disease.

There is no highly effective and safe antischistosomal drug available. All currently employed compounds have serious cardiac, renal, gastro-intestinal and even spermatogenic side-effects that seriously limit their usefulness. There is no simple answer to the questions of whether and who and how to treat; each clinical decision is influenced by many factors.

Two of the available drugs I favour are:

(a) Sodium antimony dimercaptosuccinate (Astiban or TWSB). This drug has the advantage of being administered intramuscularly in a 5-day course, but has the same effects as other antimony compounds. The standard dosage is for a total of 40 mg/kg in 5 divided injections.

(b) Niridazole (Ambilhar) is an orally administered nitrothiazole derivative that is better tolerated than any other schistosomicidal drug, but, regrettably, it is not as effective in *S. mansoni* infections as in urinary schistosomiasis. The standard regimen is 25/kg for 5 days, but 7- and 10-day courses are also employed.

Other compounds include intravenous sodium or potassium anti-mony tartrate, intramuscular stibophen or Fuadin, and the organo-phosphorous derivations such as Dipterix. I do not use any of these routinely, and I believe their toxicity outweighs their potential benefit. Because of the clear experimental demonstration of the immunological basis for granuloma formation in schistosomiasis, it is probable that pharmacological or alternative methods to suppress granuloma forma-tion will be a useful addition to specific chemotherapy. This approach has not yet been perfected.

Since all of the drugs which are currently used have their primary effect on the adult worm, eggs may be found in the stool for 6 to 8 weeks after initial therapy. Patients should be considered 'cured' only when stool and/or rectal biopsy specimens remain negative for *S. mansoni* after quarterly examinations for 1 year. Therapeutic measures such as portacaval anastomosis, cord decompression or digitalization may, of course, be useful adjuncts to the antischistosomal drugs in selected cases. Patients who are visiting areas where schistosomiasis is endemic should be advised to avoid swimming or wading in freshwater ponds or drinking the water. Worried patients in areas such as New York should be reassured that transmission of schistosomiasis from the large Latin American reservoir cannot occur, since the intermediate snail vectors do not migrate from the tropics.

BIBLIOGRAPHY

Cahill, K. (ed.). Schistosomiasis—A Symposium. *Bull. N.Y. Acad. Med.* **44,** 227–331, 1968.

Mostofoi, F. (ed.). *Bilharziasis.* New York, Springer-Verlag, 1967.

Jordan, P., and Webbe, G. *Human Schistosomiasis.* London, Heinemann, 1969.

Smithers, S. The Immunology of Schistosomiasis. *Adv. Parasitol.* **7,** 41, 1969.

Warren, K. F., and Newill, V. A. *Schistosomiasis: A Bibliography of the World's Literature from 1852 to 1962.* 2 vol., Cleveland, Press of Western Reserve University, 1967.

13 Other Schistosomal Infections

The other two main schistosomal infections of man are urinary schistosomiasis and Oriental schistosomiasis.

SCHISTOSOMA HAEMATOBIUM INFECTIONS

Urinary schistosomiasis (bilharziasis), caused by the parasite *Schistoma haematobium*, affects over 100 million people in Africa and the Middle East. Recent irrigation projects such as the Aswan Dam in the heavily infested waters of the Nile Valley have extended the geographic distribution of infected snail hosts, and several million new infections have been diagnosed in the past decade in Egypt alone. It has recently been estimated that over 15 million Egyptians are infected with *S. haematobium*, and their annual economic loss due to the parasitic disease is almost 600 million dollars.

Pathological features. The life cycle of the parasite is similar to that described previously for *S. mansoni*. The only major differences are that the adult worms lie primarily in vesical rather than mesenteric vessels, that the eggs are excreted in the urine rather than in the stool, and that the snail hosts are distinct. Pathological changes during the period of parasitic penetration, migration and maturation are also comparable with those described for *S. mansoni*.

The primary pathological changes of urinary schistosomiasis are in the vesical mucosa and submucosa. Characteristic reactions in the bilharzial bladder include the following: in the submucosa, abscess formation; in the mucosa, thickening, ulceration, calcification, pseudo-

103

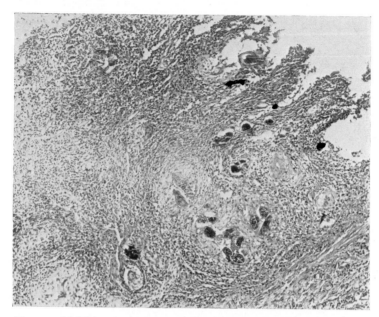

Fig. 41.   Multiple calcified *Schistosoma haematobium* in a biopsy of the bladder wall. The tissue is infiltrated with leukocytes and shows early granuloma formation.

tubercle and polyp and papilloma formation, with villous cystitis and squamous metaplasia. Foreign-body reaction with leukocytic infiltration (Fig. 41) and superimposed bacterial infection are common. Chronic bilharzial changes include obstruction of the ureteral orifices with resultant hydroureter and hydronephrosis, vesical and urethral fistulas, and anaplasia of the mucosa.

The most serious sequel of urinary schistosomiasis is the evolution of bladder cancer. Vesical carcinoma is extremely rare in the United States, accounting for less than 1 per cent of all cancers. On the other hand, in Egypt, where *S. haematobium* was demonstrable in 40 per cent of autopsies in a general survey, bladder neoplasms are the tumours most commonly seen. Underlying bilharzial infection was found in 83 per cent of all vesical cancers in this survey. Squamous cell carcinoma is the type which is most commonly encountered, correlating well with the high incidence of squamous metaplasia. Experimental studies have incriminated chronic irritation by the eggs and the toxic secretions of the parasite as causative factors, but the exact pathogenesis is undetermined.

Clinical features. The early signs and symptoms of bilharziasis are similar to those described for *S. mansoni* infection. Symptoms referable

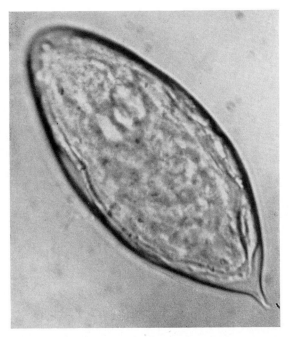

Fig. 42. High-power view of an *S. haematobium* ovum, with the typical terminal spine visible.

to vesical involvement occur in only a small percentage of infected patients. Urgency and frequency of urination, mild dysuria or terminal haematuria are often the earliest indications. Gross, persistent haematuria, urinary retention, severe dysuria, incontinence and fistulous formation are seen in advanced disease.

Diagnosis. The identification of the terminally spined eggs of *S. haematobium* is necessary for confirmation of bilharziasis (Fig. 42). Cystoscopy may reveal the characteristic mucosal changes described, and biopsy of these areas will often reveal *S. haematobium* ova in large numbers. Gross calcification of the bladder is a common X-ray finding (Fig. 43) in advanced cases, and intravenous pyelography may provide added evidence of secondary renal damage. Aberrant localization of eggs occurs in urinary schistosomiasis; they may be found in the sputum of patients with anomalous vascular shunts or severe pulmonary hypertension; they are occasionally detected in biopsy sections of the skin, particularly in the inguinal area (Fig. 44), the eye and the brain. Skin tests, complement-fixation and other immunologically based procedures are of the same value as in *S. mansoni* infections.

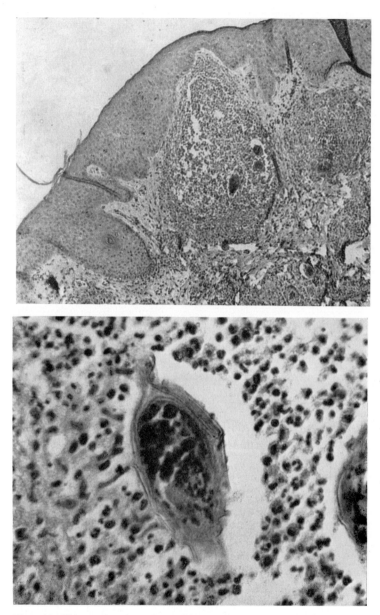

Fig. 44. Skin section in a boy with cutaneous schistosomiasis, showing, *bottom*, the characteristic *S. haematobium* morphology.

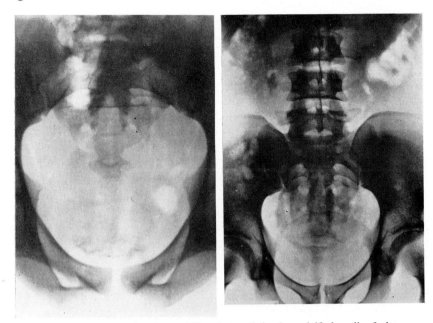

Fig. 43. Advanced urinary bilharziasis. *Left*, the calcified wall of the bladder, when it is contracted, appears as 'crumpled paper'. *Right*, the bladder, when it is dilated with urine, has been likened to a fetal head.

Treatment. Ambilhar is highly effective and is my choice for the chemotherapy of *S. haematobium* infections. In general, urinary schistosomiasis responds more readily to antibilharzial drugs than is the case with either *S. mansoni* or *S. japonicum*. All the compounds listed in the preceding chapter are feasible alternatives.

The bilharzial tubercle on the bladder wall disappears or diminishes after therapy, and post-therapy cystoscopy may reveal only pallor or residual scarring. Urological surgical treatment is often indicated in the patient with advanced disease. Dilatation of constricted ureters is helpful, and excision of stenotic orifices may be necessary, Cystotomy or ileocystoplasty may be useful in patients with contracted, calcific bladders. Repair of fistulas is imperative, and antibiotic therapy for superimposed bacterial infection is a further necessary adjunct.

SCHISTOSOMA JAPONICUM INFECTIONS

The global incidence of Oriental schistosomiasis, caused by *S. japonicum*, cannot be determined today with accuracy. It is estimated that 30 million people are infected, but in recent years there have been few valid statistics available from the area of highest incidence, the Yangtze Valley in China. Endemic foci exist in Formosa, Japan and the Philippines, Thailand and Laos. Despite this limited distribution, the potential danger of the parasite can be demonstrated by the fact that at least 1,500 American soldiers during World War II were known to be infected within a period of 6 months on the island of Leyte.

Pathological features. The life cycle of *S. japonicum* is similar to that described for *S. mansoni* except that a specific intermediate snail vector exists, and, most importantly, other mammals may serve as definitive hosts. The adult worms lie in the mesenteric vessels, and the female *S. japonicum* produces about 11 times as many eggs as her *mansoni* counterpart.

The pathogenesis of the lesions is the same for both infections, but the histological changes are correspondingly more severe in Oriental schistosomiasis. Submucosal abscess formation is more extensive, mucosal proliferation greater, and polyp formation, fibrotic strictures, fissures and prolapse are more common. Hepatosplenic damage is also more severe, in both the acute and the chronic stages. Presinusoidal and postsinusoidal hypertension become marked in untreated cases, with resultant variceal formation and ascites. The central nervous system is involved in 2·5 per cent of cases. The typical lesion is an expanding granulomatous tumour with a necrotic centre and a giant-cell border. There may be pressure atrophy of surrounding brain tissue. Other unusual sites of involvement are the eye, the heart and the skin.

Clinical features. Unlike patients with the other two schistosomal infections, the majority (80 to 90 per cent) with an initial infection with *S. japonicum* have a marked clinical reaction. Fever, chills, abdominal pain, diarrhoea, weight loss, a hacking, nonproductive cough, urticaria, malaise, anorexia, tender hepatosplenomegaly (in 90 per cent), diffuse moist rales and a stiff neck are common signs and symptoms during the acute phase of egg deposition, which occurs about 1 month after exposure. Chronic features of the disease include haematemesis, ascites, anaemia and other evidence of terminal liver failure.

Diagnosis. The identification of the *S. japonicum* ova is the surest way to confirm a diagnosis of Oriental schistosomiasis. During the early phase of generalized symptoms, this is not a major problem, for eggs are being excreted in great numbers. If one searches in the mucus or a bloodstained section of the stool or uses a simple water-concentrating technique, eggs can be found quickly in over 90 per cent of infected patients. After inadequate therapy or in the chronic phase the demonstration of eggs is much more difficult. Five times as many stool examinations are required to detect infected patients, and much more patience and experience is required of the parasitologist. The use of rectal snips, mucus smears and liver biopsies will increase the positive yield, as noted in *S. mansoni* infections. The *S. japonicum* eggs are about one third smaller than those of the other schistosomes and have a minute lateral spine.

Serological tests are useful, though false positive and false negative results do occur occasionally. However, because of the severe natural history of this disease and the poor prognosis of untreated cases, a positive serological result in a patient with a history of exposure and characteristic clinical symptoms, despite negative results of stool examination, is a sufficient basis for treatment in this variety of schistosomiasis. Eosinophilia is invariably present in the acute phase but may be absent in the chronic stage. Sigmoidoscopy reveals abnormalities in the large majority of untreated patients, with over two thirds revealing characteristic elevated, firm yellow nodules in the rectosigmoid; however, a barium enema examination is usually normal. Cerebrospinal fluid was found to be abnormal in a third of the soldiers with neurological lesions.

Treatment. The high morbidity and high mortality of Oriental schistosomiasis can be prevented by early and adequate therapy. Because of the serious complications in untreated cases, treatment in this variety of schistosomiasis can be instituted on clinical plus immunological evidence, even if eggs cannot be detected. Despite the ominous prognosis that most textbooks state is typical, there was not a single fatality after a proper regimen of diagnosis and drug dosage had been initiated in the large military group infected on Leyte. Specific treatment will even alleviate symptoms of neurological lesions but will not alter the outcome if damage caused by chronic liver involvement is evident.

Ambilhar, Astiban and Fuadin are not as effective against *S. japonicum* as against the other two schistosomes. Viable eggs will persist after therapy in 50 per cent of patients. The antimony compound, tartar emetic, is the drug of choice and should be administered intravenously. A total of 2·22 g in a 0·5 per cent solution (444 ml) should be injected on alternate days over a period of 35 days, with an initial dose of 8 ml and an average one of 28 ml. Toxic reactions, including arthralgias, coughing paroxysms, nausea, vomiting and conjunctivitis, occur in a high percentage of patients, and the regimen should be undertaken only with the patient under hospital observation. Necrosis of tissue may occur if the drug extravasates into the perivascular tissue. Serious toxic reactions such as cardiac arrhythmias and hypotension are rare if administration is not too rapid and the dosage is not exceeded. Neverthe-less, cardiac disease is a relative contraindication, as is advanced hepatic decompensation.

Neurosurgical treatment is indicated for schistosomal brain lesions, and portacaval anastomosis may alleviate variceal bleeding in patients with advanced cirrhosis.

RARE SCHISTOSOMAL INFECTIONS

Man may serve as an abnormal host to a wide variety of schistosomes. At least 20 different species have been reported to cause transient dermatitis, and several have caused vesical and intestinal symptoms in isolated cases.

BIBLIOGRAPHY

Honey, R., and Gelfand, M. *The Urological Aspects of Bilharziasis in Rhodesia.* Edinburgh, Livingstone, 1960.
Cheng, T. Schistosomiasis in Mainland China. *Am. J. trop. Med. Hyg.* **20,** 26, 1971.
Most, H., *et al.* Schistosomiasis japonica in American Military Personnel: Clinical Studies of 600 cases during the First Year after Infection. *Am. J. trop. Med.* **30,** 239, 1950.
Cahill, K., and Mofty, A. Cutaneous Lesions in Schistosomiasis. *Am. J. trop. Med. Hyg.* **13,** 800, 1964.

14   Echinococcosis

Hydatid disease, or echinococcosis, occurs in temperate and frigid climates as well as in the tropics. At the present time the highest rates of incidence are in Africa, the Middle East, Australia, New Zealand and South America. Even within the endemic zones, however, the frequency of human cases is limited to rural inhabitants living in close association with infected dogs. Hydatid disease is an occupational hazard of sheep-herders in some areas. Since cysts, once formed, remain in man, the disease is seen in the United States and Europe among immigrants from endemic areas.   Although the mortality rate is low, the mor-bidity from this disease is appreciable.

Pathological features

The causative agent of unilocular hydatid disease is the small tape-worm *Echinococcus granulosus*. Alveolar echinococcosis, a distinct entity caused by *E. multilocularis*, will be discussed briefly later. Man is an abnormal intermediate host in the life cycle of the parasite, with the sheep as the usual intermediary and the dog as the definitive host. The small adult tapeworm, consisting of only 3 to 4 proglottids, exists sym-biotically in the intestines of infected dogs. When the terminal proglottid ruptures, 500 to 1,000 eggs are excreted in the faeces. Because of a chitinous covering, the eggs may remain viable in soil for months in spite of exposure to sun and wind. When they are ingested by grazing animals, the shell is destroyed by gastric acid, and the egg hatches in the duodenum. The liberated embryo migrates through the intestinal mucosa and is carried in the vascular channels to the liver and other viscera, where the larval form develops into a cyst. The cycle is com-pleted when a dog eats the viscera of infected animals, and scolices from the cyst develop into adult tapeworms.

Man may enter the cycle, as may cattle, camels, pigs and horses, by ingesting the eggs. This occurs most commonly when children play on ground contaminated by the faeces of infected dogs. Eggs also adhere to the hair of dogs; when adults pet the animals and fail to wash, they may become infected by hand-to-mouth transmission.

Since the liver serves as the primary filter for the mesenteric venous return, the great majority of unilocular hydatid cysts are found there (Table 7). However, other organs may be involved either by primary

Table 7. Frequency of localization of solitary, unilocular hydatid cysts in various sites in man

Site	Percentage of Cases
Liver	79
Lungs	9
Muscle	6
Bone	2
Kidneys	2
Spleen	1
Brain	1

deposition or following rupture of a hepatic cyst. The development of the cyst, regardless of the site, requires many months, and, by the time symptoms first appear, years have usually elapsed.

As the cyst (Fig. 45) enlarges, the adjacent host tissue initially shows histologic evidence of both inflammation and pressure atrophy. A thick, calcified capsule eventually develops. The cyst within is composed of an external laminated layer and an inner germinal layer, with pedunculated brood capsules containing hooklets and scolices (Fig. 46). The

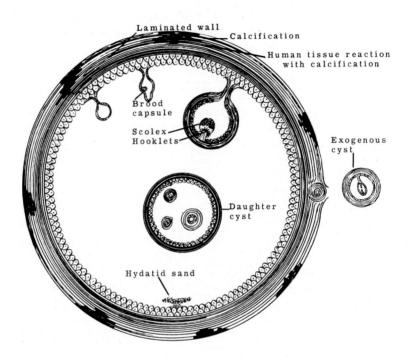

UNILOCULAR HYDATID CYST

Fig. 45. Diagrammatic representation of *Echinococcus granulosus* cyst. Microscopic details are shown in Figure 46.

stalks of these capsules may separate from the germinal layer so that daughter cysts float in the hydatid fluid. If the brood capsule or a daughter cyst ruptures, the scolices and the hooklets fall to the bottom of the cyst, forming 'hydatid sand'. Complete calcific encapsulation will prevent adequate nutrition and cause caseation of the cyst. Other complications include rupture of the cyst, secondary metastatic spread, and infection resulting in a pyogenic abscess.

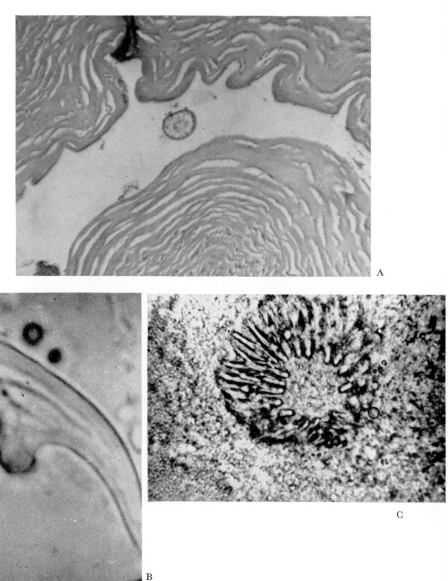

Fig. 46. A, typical scolex and laminated wall of hydatid cyst. B and C, phase photomicrographs of scraping from the inner lining of a hydatid cyst, showing, B, hooklet and, C, scolex.

Clinical features

The majority of patients with echinococcosis are asymptomatic. When clinical manifestations of the disease do occur, they are related either to the location of the cyst or to an allergic reaction to its contents. The classical triad of biliary colic, urticaria and jaundice that is associated with hydatid lesions of the liver is based on the rupture of intrahepatic cysts into the biliary tree. Pulmonary and even peri-cardiac cysts may assume significant size and yet remain clinically inapparent; in fact, many diagnoses of hydatid disease are an un-expected finding in routine X-ray of the chest and abdomen.

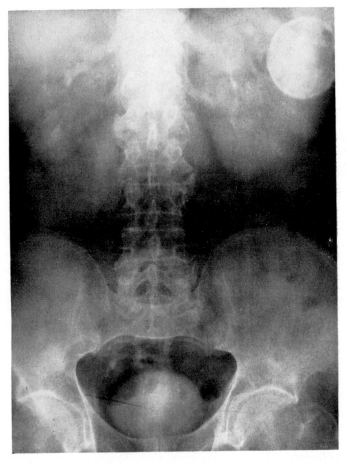

Fig. 47. Solitary splenic cyst with characteristic calcific border and areas of increased density within the cyst structure.

The physical finding of a 'hydatid thrill', attributed to movement of the daughter cysts on percussion, is neither frequent nor specific and appears, to me, to be found more in textbooks than in clinical practice. Secondary bacterial infection of cysts results in the destruction of the parasite and the production of the tender hepatomegaly and the spiking temperatures seen in patients with pyogenic liver abscesses. Because of pressure atrophy and destruction of trabeculae, hydatid cysts of bone often are manifested as pathologic fractures. Echinococcal involvement of the kidneys may cause flank pain, dysuria or haematuria. As with any slow-growing brain tumour, cerebral hydatid lesions present the pattern of focal epilepsy. Splenic cysts are rarely symptomatic (Fig. 47).

In the United States, the patients most seriously ill with hydatid disease usually present iatrogenically induced, anaphylactic reactions due to release of foreign protein in hydatid fluid at the time of unnecessary or unwise surgical intervention (Fig. 48).

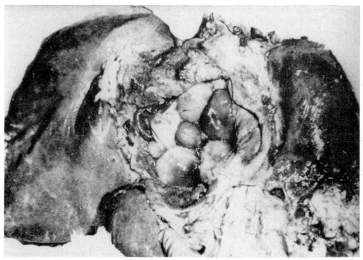

Fig. 48. Necropsy specimen of a unilocular hydatid cyst with rupture and extension into the biliary tree.

Diagnosis

In areas where echinococcosis is endemic there is little diagnostic challenge in confirming the suspicion of hydatid disease. There is a characteristic X-ray picture, and highly specific skin and serological tests are available. Since man is an abnormal intermediate host and adult worms do not develop, it is obvious that eggs cannot be found in human faeces.

The Casoni skin test, an intracutaneous injection of 0·1 ml of echinococcal antigen, shows a positive reaction in approximately 80 per cent of patients with hydatid disease. There is an immediate (15-minute flare) reaction and a delayed (12-hour indurated wheal) reaction. The Casoni test reaction will remain positive even years after surgical removal of a hydatid cyst. Many serological tests are available for the diagnosis of hydatid disease. The most reliable are the haemagglutination and the bentonite flocculation tests; in combination they are positive in over 95 per cent of patients with echinococcosis. Although not specific, eosinophilia, frequently in the range of 40 to 50 per cent, is common.

Because of calcification in the reactive host tissue surrounding the lesion, pathognomonic X-ray patterns of various hydatid lesions are described. If the cyst is in the liver, the right side of the diaphragm may be raised and fixed while the hepatic flexure of the colon is displaced downward. Displacement of adjacent structures is also common in other viscera. Bone involvement may be manifested as irregular areas of absorption or rarefaction throughout the cancellous portion.

The definitive diagnostic test is the demonstration of the hooklets and the scolices within the laminated cyst wall. This may be accomplished by surgical exploration and excision but never by exploratory percutaneous aspiration, a procedure that can result in the spread of the hydatid lesions as well as in severe allergic reactions.

Treatment

Surgical excision of accessible cysts is the sole treatment for hydatid disease. Unnecessary surgical intervention is, however, responsible for most fatalities in those with well-calcified hydatid cysts, as seen in the older immigrant population in the United States. The decision whether to remove or leave alone a well-calcified, asymptomatic cyst is an individual clinical one. The possibility of hydatid disease should be considered in the differential diagnosis of cystic or space-occupying masses in those from endemic areas, but the confirmation of diagnosis alone is not an adequate basis for surgical intervention.

If surgery is considered desirable, then, after adequate exposure and careful packing off of surrounding tissue, the cyst wall should be punctured by a sterile needle, and 50 to 100 ml of hydatid fluid should be withdrawn if possible. Then 5 to 10 ml of a 10 per cent formalin solution should be injected through the same needle and a 20-minute period allowed for destruction of the parasite before further manipulation. This tedious manoeuvre is essential to prevent severe allergic reactions and the spread of echinococcosis by leakage of the cyst contents. Excision should include the calcific reactive host tissue as well as the entire cyst lining. There is no effective chemotherapeutic agent for hydatid disease, and radiation therapy is useless.

ALVEOLAR HYDATID DISEASE

The general term echinococcosis also includes alveolar hydatid disease, which is caused by *E. multilocularis*, a parasite that is anatomically and epidemiologically distinct from *E. granulosus*; it is found in wolves, foxes and mice in the more frigid portions of Alaska, Russia and the Alps. Man is an abnormal intermediate host to the destructive larval stage. Alveolar hydatid disease differs from the unilocular variety in that the lesion produced by *E. multilocularis* is an infiltrative, neoplastic-like invasion, with poorly defined borders. The liver and the lung are most commonly involved, and the clinical manifestations are those expected from chronic destruction of these organs. Casoni and complement-fixation tests are unreliable, and no characteristic X-ray picture is seen. Treatment is by surgical excision, if possible. The prognosis is poor.

BIBLIOGRAPHY

Powers, L., and Churchill, C.   *Bibliography of Echinococcosis with Selected Abstracts.*   Beirut, Lebanon, American University of Beirut Press, 1960.
Schantz, P., and Schwabe, C.   Worldwide Status of Hydatid Disease Control.   *J. Am. vet. med. Ass.* **155,** 2104, 1969.
Williams, J., *et al*.   Current Prevalence and Distribution of Hydatidosis.   *Am. J. trop. Med. Hyg.* **20,** 224, 1971.

15   More Trematode and Cestode Infections

TREMATODE INFECTIONS

The most important trematodes of man, the schistosomes, have already been considered. Other trematodes or flukes are also of major medical significance, especially in the Far East, as parasites of the human liver, lung and intestinal tract. The life cycles of trematodes, exclusive of the schistosomes, are similar: an egg, excreted by the definitive host (e.g. man), develops through sporocyst and redia stages in the hepato-pancreas of specific snail hosts; cercariae emerge from the snail and encyst as metacercariae in fish, crustaceans or water plants; human disease follows the ingestion of infective second intermediate hosts.

The parasite excysts in the human duodenum and reaches adult size in from 1 to 6 weeks. The flukes of man are hermaphroditic, and production and excretion of ova renew the life cycle. The identification of adult flukes is based on the morphology of gut, testes, yolk glands and suckers. These details, which are available in any text of parasitology, are rarely important to the diagnostician and will not be repeated here. On the other hand, knowledge of the characteristic shapes of ova is essential to anyone attempting stool examination.

Clonorchiasis. The Chinese liver fluke, *Clonorchis sinensis*, is a frequent parasite of man throughout the Far East. Clonorchiasis is commonly diagnosed in communities with populations of Oriental origin. Man becomes infected by eating raw or undercooked freshwater fish harbouring metacercaria of *C. sinensis*.

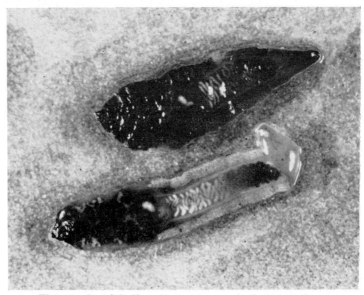

Fig. 49. An adult *Clonorchis sinensis* worm in the human liver.

In heavy or repeated infections, low-grade fever, eosinophilia, diarrhoea and evidence of hepatobiliary damage occur. Reaction to the parasite results in hyperplasia and adenomatous proliferation (Fig. 49) of the epithelial lining of bile capillaries. Cholangitis, periductal fibrosis, hepatitis, centrolobular cirrhosis with jaundice, ascites and hepatomegaly may result from severe infections.

In light or moderate infections Strauss has noted that Caucasians with clonorchiasis complain of many more symptoms than do their stoical Oriental counterparts; most of the symptoms cited cannot be attributed with confidence to *C. sinensis*.

Diagnosis is made by visualizing operculated, lemon-shaped eggs (Fig. 50) in faecal preparations. There is no effective treatment for

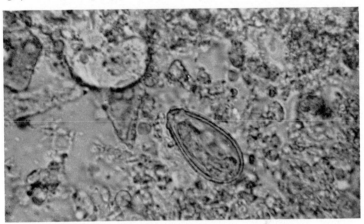

Fig. 50.   High-power view of a *C. sinensis* egg.

clonorchiasis. The most popular therapeutic regimen today is $\frac{1}{2}$ g of chloroquine phosphate daily for 2 months. Cure rates are less than 75 per cent; furthermore, one third of the 'cured' cases have positive stool examinations within a year.

Other liver flukes. Less important liver flukes which infect man include *Opisthorchis felineus*, *O. viverrini*, *Dicrocelium dendriticum*, *Fasciola gigantica* and *F. hepatica*. The last-named fluke is unique in that water-cress serves as its second intermediate host. Though human cases are common in France, England and Latin America, no indigenous cose of fascioliasis has been described in the United States.

Paragonimiasis. *Paragonimus westermani* is the sole pulmonary fluke of man. Throughout the Orient, and particularly in South Korea, paragonimiasis is prevalent. When infective eggs are expectorated into snail-laden water, a developmental cycle similar to that described for *C. sinensis* commences. Cercariae, liberated from the snails, penetrate crabs or crayfish, and man acquires the disease by eating these crusta-ceans uncooked. The fluke excysts in the human duodenum, burrows through the gut wall into the liver, and matures in the lungs.

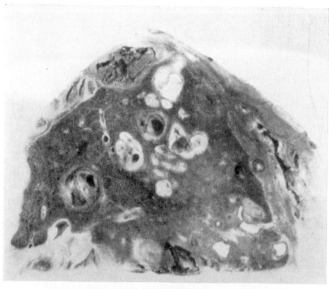

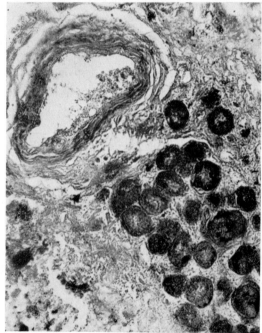

Fig. 51. *Top,* multiple cysts in the lung of a Korean with *Paragonimus wester-mani* infection. *Bottom,* histological section demonstrating communication of a bronchiole with the cyst.

The young *Paragonimus* stimulates eosinophilic and fibrotic reactions in the bronchioles, and, as the parasite grows, characteristic cysts concentrated along the pleural surface of the lung (Fig. 51) develop. Communication of cysts with bronchioles permits the discharge of eggs in purulent, blood-tinged sputum. Patients experience cough, pleuritic pain, low-grade fever, weight loss and malaise. The clinical syndrome is not specific and must be differentiated from tuberculosis, bronchiectasis and pneumonia. Aberrant localization of *Paragonimus* produces bizarre clinical patterns; cerebral lesions may produce epileptic seizures, haemiplegia, paresis and ocular disturbances. Suppurative cysts in the liver, the spleen, the mesentery and the intestine have been reported sites of abdominal paragonimiasis.

Diagnosis is based on visualization of ova of *P. westermani* in sputum or faeces. Eosinophilia is usually present. The chemotherapy of paragonimiasis is in a state of flux. Chloroquine, emetine and antimony compounds have been in vogue at various times, but none was consistently effective. Korean investigators have reported a high cure rate following intramuscular administration of Bithionol in a dose of 30 mg per kg on alternate days for 10 days. Occasionally, surgical removal of localized cysts is possible.

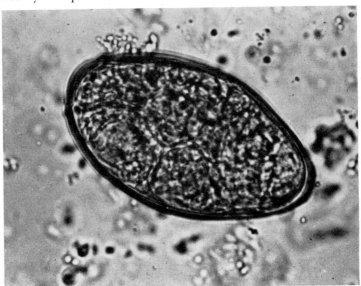

Fig. 52. Oil-immersion view of *Heterophyes heterophyes* egg.

Intestinal flukes. Intestinal flukes rarely produce symptoms in man. Even a heavy parasitic burden of *Heterophyes heterophyes* or

Metagonimus yokogawai, two common intestinal flukes in Africa and Asia, is associated only with mild diarrhoea. *Fasciola buski*, the other major trematode of the human gut, can cause epigastric pain, diarrhoea and even oedema and anasarca, though this syndrome occurs more frequently in textbooks than in reality. The metacercariae of *H. heterophyes* and *M. yokogawai* encyst in freshwater fish; those of *F. buski* lodge in waternut plants. Man acquires the diseases by eating undercooked, infective items.

Diagnosis of these infections is made by detecting characteristic ova in stool examinations (Fig. 52). Treatment of heterophyiasis and metagonimiasis with tetrachlorethylene is effective; the regimen outlined for hookworm should be followed. Fasciolopsiasis can be cured by a single oral dose of hexylresorcinol (1 g) followed 2 hours later by a purgative.

CESTODE INFECTIONS

The cestodes, or tapeworms, of man are present throughout the world. None of these helminths exists solely in the tropics, and several of the class are prevalent only in frigid climates. An extraintestinal tapeworm infection, echinococcosis, has already been described in detail. To complete an adequate outline of parasitic diseases and allow for the proper recognition and interpretation of stool ova, a brief discussion of other tapeworm infections is provided here.

Taeniasis saginata. The beef tapeworm, *Taenia saginata*, is a flat, hermaphroditic worm from 10 to 15 feet long and is composed of several thousand segments, or proglottids. Each proglottid contains testes and an ovary; fertilization occurs between adjacent segments. Gravid terminal segments are longer than they are broad and contain a uterus with more than 13 lateral branches (Fig. 53). Gravid proglottids may be defecated intact, or they may rupture within the large bowel, and taenia eggs (Fig. 54) are then excreted. Cattle are the most important intermediate hosts and man is the only definitive host.

Human infection follows the ingestion of raw or undercooked beef containing an invaginated larval form of the parasite, a cysticercus bovis. The larva evaginates in the duodenum, the scolex attaches to the jejunum, and the worm grows gradually, segment by segment, down the small intestine.

Human disease is often asymptomatic and, in spite of the large size of the cestode, bowel disturbances are rarely prominent. Vague abdominal pains and nonspecific nervous reactions often accompany taeniasis. A moderate eosinophilia is common.

Diagnosis depends on the finding of a taenia egg and/or a gravid proglottid. The drug of choice is niclosamide (Yomesan). This medication is taken as a single course with four tablets, well chewed, followed

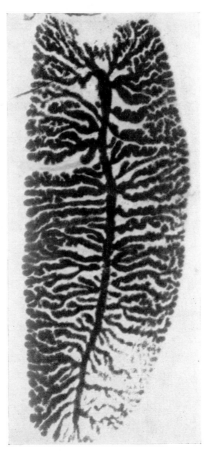

Fig. 53.   Gravid segment of *Taenia saginata*. The lateral uterine branches are outlined with India ink.

by water. Since the drug destroys the parasite, it is not necessary to indulge in a tedious search for the scolex in masses of faeces and disintegrating worms, as the case with Atabrine. Treatment with a single oral dose of quinacrine hydrochloride (Atabrine or mepacrine) (0·5 to 1·0 g) after a 12-hour fast is curative in about 75 per cent of patients. The use of a purgative 2 hours after medication assists in freeing the scolex from the gut wall. In refractory cases, administration of the drug by duodenal intubation is sometimes helpful. Extract of male fern is an alternative and equally effective vermifuge. It is essential to

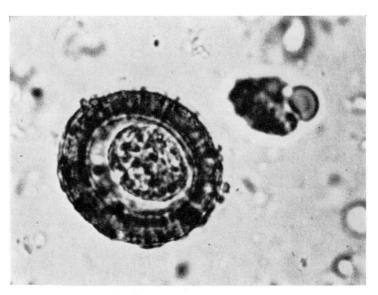

Fig. 54.   High-power view of a taenia egg.

identify the scolex in faecal examination before concluding that treatment with quinacrine or male fern was successful.

Taeniasis solium. Both the adult and the larval forms of the pork tapeworm, *T. solium*, parasitize man. The adult worm lives in the small intestine; it can be differentiated from *T. saginata* by the elevated rostellum with 2 rows of hooks on the scolex and by gravid proglottids with less than 13 lateral branches. The eggs of beef tapeworms and those of pork tapeworms are indistinguishable.

Man can serve both as an intermediate host and as the definitive host of *T. solium*. If an egg (instead of the usual larval cyst) is ingested or is regurgitated into the stomach during vomiting, an oncosphere is liberated which penetrates the gut wall and can be circulated anywhere in the body. Skin, muscles and brain are most commonly invaded, but only with involvement of the brain are symptoms common. As the larval form invaginates and the resultant cyst (cysticercus cellulosa) expands, several syndromes occur, depending on the number and the site of the lesions. Cysts in the cerebral substance are associated with epilepsy; cysts in the fourth ventricle can produce intermittent blockage of the aqueduct of Sylvius (Brunn's syndrome).

Diagnosis of cysticercus cerebri may be made by X-ray visualization of calcified cysts or by histology at operation or postmortem examination. Moderate eosinophilia and a positive result from complement-fixation tests on cerebrospinal fluid provide supportive evidence. Surgical removal of ventricular cysts is curative; operative intervention is impossible when multiple cysts stud the brain. Chemotherapy for cysticercosis is ineffective. Yomesan is the drug of choice for pork tapeworm infestation.

Hymenolepis nana. The dwarf tapeworm uses man as both intermediate and definitive host. The parasite, a small cestode with a hooked scolex, produces eggs within the human intestine. Eggs (Fig. 55) are infective as soon as they are passed in the stool, and trans-

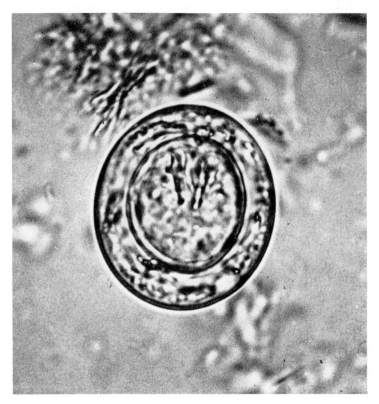

Fig. 55. High-power view of *Hymenolepis nana* egg.

mission is via the anal–oral route. Infection is usually asymptomatic. Treatment with Yomesan, as outlined for taeniasis, is effective.

Diphyllobothrium latum. This parasite is more common in the northern temperate climates than in the tropics or the subtropics. Freshwater lake areas of Scandinavia and the north-central United States have long been endemic zones, though the disease can occur whenever this cestode's intermediate host, freshwater fish, is transported and eaten raw. Jewish housewives savouring uncooked gefilte fish account for many infections. Despite its enormous size, occasionally exceeding 30 feet in length, *D. latum* rarely produces gastrointestinal symptoms. The worm is probably best known for its role as an exotic cause of megaloblastic anaemia. When the scolex is attached high up in the small intestine, the parasite can compete with man for available Vitamin B_{12}. Yomesan is an effective vermifuge for *D. latum* infection. Parenteral B_{12} is necessary if megaloblastic anaemia is present.

BIBLIOGRAPHY

Yobogawa, M.   Paragonimus and Paragonimiasis.   *Adv. Parasitol.* **7,** 375, 1969.
Komiya, Y.   Clonorchis and Clonorchiasis.   *Adv. Parasitol.* **4,** 53, 1966.
Bonsdoroff, B. von.   *D. latum* as a Cause of Pernicious Anemia.   *Expl Parasit.* **5,** 207, 1956.
Strauss, W.   Clinical Manifestations of Clonorchiasis: a Controlled Study of 105 Cases.   *Am. J. trop. Med. Hyg.* **11,** 625, 1962.

III BACTERIAL DISEASES

---

16 Leprosy

Leprosy has been known since antiquity. The Egyptians noted it among their slaves thirteen hundred years before Christ. Confucius mentions it, as do the early Vedic physicians of India. The Old Testament refers to lepers, and a famous parable in the New Testament describes a well-organized system of community isolation against leprous persons. It is likely that many unrelated dermatologic lesions were considered leprous in biblical times. The disease was apparently very prevalent in Europe during the Middle Ages but did not exist in the Americas before the advent of the white man in the fifteenth century. The incidence in North America was later markedly increased by the importation of infected slaves from areas of Africa where leprosy was endemic.

The cause of leprosy was unknown to the ancients. It was believed to be a punishment of God, and patients with leprosy were ostracized more for religious and aesthetic reasons than as a public health measure. Later, it was thought to be a hereditary disease, and possibly a venereal one. Linnaeus attributed it to eating fish contaminated with nematodes. In the nineteenth century Jonathan Hutchinson expounded the fish theory, and in the first edition of Osler's textbook this possibility is strongly considered. As late as 1908 Balfour wrote in his *Recent Advances in Tropical Medicine* that 'one notes the tendency to attribute the disease in the first instance to the bites of insects'.

The controversy as to the cause of leprosy has persisted into the twentieth century even though in 1874 a Norwegian physician, Gerhard Hansen, described a bacillus consistently found in the nodules of patients with leprosy. Although his description preceded Koch's discovery of the tubercle bacillus by 8 years, final proof of the aetiological significance of *Mycobacterium leprae* is yet to come. For Koch's postulates have yet to be fulfilled: the organism has neither been successfully cultured nor has it been transmitted experimentally to animals.

Epidemiological aspects

Because of the gaps in our knowledge of the infectivity of *M. leprae*, the epidemiology of leprosy is based more on clinical impressions and deductions than on bacteriological or pathological studies. Man is generally considered the sole source of the disease. Rat leprosy is a distinct entity, and there is no convincing evidence that this variety is contagious to man. As already noted, there has been only very limited success in the frequent attempts at transmitting human leprosy to animals. Recently, *M. leprae* have been inoculated into and maintained in the footpads of mice. However, this modest demonstration of bacteria multiplication, and the eventual transmission of organisms and infection to subsequent animal models, must still be considered a research technique, and not yet a practical laboratory aid to the clinician. The routine *in vitro* cultivation of aetiological organisms is not yet available for the leprologist.

The mode of transmission of leprosy from man to man is still a topic of debate among leprologists. The bacilli are commonly believed to enter either via the nasal mucous membranes or through the skin. The factors which have been considered most important in determining infectivity are: (1) the age of the patient at exposure, (2) the closeness of contact, (3) the extent of infection, and (4) individual susceptibility.

The high childhood incidence which has been found in many studies is probably due to the intimate contact that infants have with lepromatous adults. Although leprosy has been detected in infants as young as 4 months, the average age of onset in childhood is 3 years. Estimates of the incubation period of leprosy usually range from 1 to 20 years. In the meagreness of our knowledge of the clinical, the bacteriological and the pathological course in the incubational phase of leprosy lies the primary reason for the failures of international control and eradication programmes.

Family and community studies in Latin America, Africa, India and the Philippines show an infection rate 8 to 10 times above normal for patients in contact with known lepromatous persons. The risk is less, but still increased, if contact is with persons who have tuberculoid leprosy. The difference in the contagiousness of these two types of leprosy is directly related to the number of *M. leprae* bacilli present. Enormous numbers can be found in lepromatous nodules, whereas only a few, or none, are seen in scrapings from or biopsies of tuberculoid lesions. Although prolonged and intimate contact with leprosy is of epidemiological significance insofar as the extent of infection and reinfection is concerned, it is not essential for the transmission of the

128

disease. I can well recall a patient whose only exposure to leprosy had been a very brief visit to North Africa during the war and who slowly developed classical lepromatous leprosy.

For a decade and a half this man had lived and worked, a stoical individual in a normal, unattentive community, with lepromatous leprosy. The physical signs of leprosy, though marked, had evolved so gradually that the patient, his neighbours and the local physicians failed to recognize the disease. The extremely short exposure to infection, the onset of signs in late middle age in an isolated village and the tragedy of delayed diagnosis in this patient all re-emphasize the need to obtain an adequate travel history from patients and, at least, to consider tropical diseases in differential diagnoses in temperate climates.

Estimates of the number of patients with leprosy in the world today vary between 5 and 10 million persons. The highest incidence rates are in Central Africa, Asia and, in the Americas, in Brazil, Colombia, Venezuela and the West Indies. In the temperate zones there remain several small foci of the disease; most are self-limiting, and the only ones of any importance are in the Baltic States and in Spain and Portugal.

Pathological and clinical features

The interpretation of any article about clinical leprosy depends on a knowledge of the classification used. During the past 50 years at least a dozen subdivisions have been in vogue at various times. Today the World Health Organization recommends only two main categories, the lepromatous and the tuberculoid. This classification is based on histological, bacteriological, immunological and clinical criteria (Table 8).

Table 8.   Points differentiating the main types of leprosy

Lepromatous	Tuberculoid
Diffuse lesions; poorly defined borders	Granulomatous lesions; well-defined borders
No anhidrosis	Anhidrosis
Symmetrical lesions	Asymmetrical lesions
Sensory loss variable	Sensory loss invariable
M. leprae abundant	M. leprae rare
Lepromin (Mitsuda–Rost reaction) negative	Lepromin (Mitsuda–Rost reaction) positive
Wassermann reaction often positive (false)	Wassermann reaction negative
Infectivity greater	Infectivity less

Very early cases may be detected in an indeterminate stage before evolving into one of the main types. There are also a large number of

129

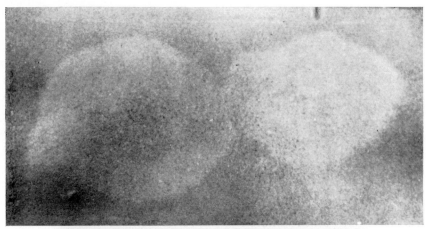

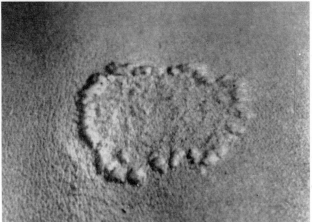

Fig. 56. Tuberculoid leprosy, often misdiagnosed as vitiligo and ringworm. The maculo-anaesthetic lesion, *top*, is flat, discrete, hypopigmented and insensitive, and may progress to an infiltrated area with raised borders, *bottom*. Scrapings of these lesions for *Mycobacterium leprae* frequently show negative findings, but biopsy will be characteristic.

cases that do not fit strictly under either main heading and are grouped as intermediate or dimorphous types.

Numbness may precede all other symptoms, and anaesthesia is the cardinal sign of leprosy. The earliest visible lesion is a flat, hypopigmented macule ranging from 0·5 to 3 cm in diameter (Fig. 56), with associated sensory loss over the central area. The resistance of the host determines what type of leprosy, if any, evolves. When host resistance is high, the skin lesion is transient, and the disease regresses completely.

In the remaining cases the *M. leprae* will spread initially in the axonal spaces of the peripheral nerves. In the tuberculoid variety there is a coalescence of epitheloid cells, inflammatory cells and lymphocytes in the dermatomes involved. As the disease progresses, the nerves gradually thicken and become palpable cords especially noticeable in the neck and the forearms. Anhidrosis is common, as, in later stages, are facial paralyses, drop foot, claw hands, lagophthalmos, bone changes and deep trophic nerve ulcers. The terminal phalanges are the osseous structures most involved, because the nutritional blood supply to the bone is impaired by the damage to the vascular nerve supply, and surface anaesthesia exposes the fingertips and the toes to multiple, unrecognized trauma and destruction (Fig. 57).

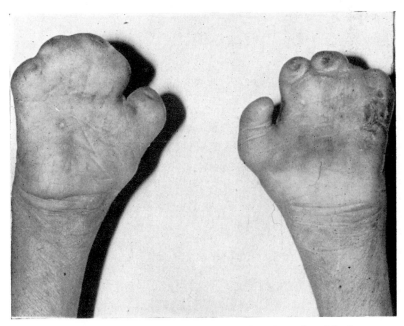

Fig. 57.   Gross deformity of the hands with complete absorption of the fingers.

Characteristic tubercles may also be found in biopsies of skin, lymph nodes and liver. Another serious, if rare, complication of tuberculoid leprosy is blindness caused by ulcerations of the cornea from lagophthalmos and unrecognized trauma to a desensitized eye. However, remission of many of the clinical manifestations of tuberculoid leprosy is frequent in patients with adequate defence mechanisms.

When host resistance is low following introduction of the *M. leprae*

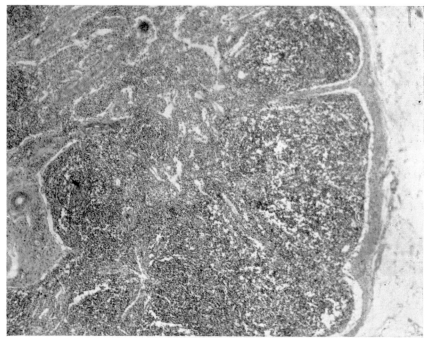

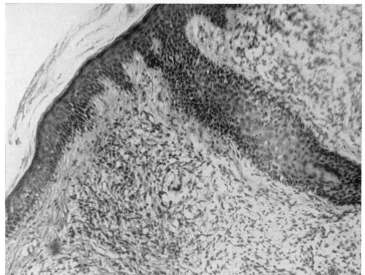

Fig. 58. *Top*, tuberculoid lesion with marked round-cell infiltration and giant-cell formation; there is no free subepidermal zone. *Bottom*, a nodular leproma, with foamy cells containing many *M. leprae* bacilli and with a clear subepidermal zone.

into the axonal spaces, massive multiplication of the bacilli occurs. The end-result is lepromatous leprosy. The incipient lesion in this type is usually a diffuse, symmetrical, macular eruption which, unlike the tuberculoid variety, has poorly defined borders and is moist. Histologically, the full-blown lepromatous lesion can be differentiated easily from the tuberculoid section. Although the earliest pathological changes in the fine sensory nerve fibres are not as striking as the granulomatous destruction in the tuberculoid type, almost all other pathological changes are more extensive. *M. leprae* abound on biopsy, and skin sections reveal marked infiltration, with plasma and reticuloendothelial cells. These cells tend to pile up in the superficial dermis, causing the typical nodules of leprosy (Fig. 58). On the face the nodules become concentrated in the intercilium and on the cheeks, the earlobes, and the jaw. There is a loss of eyebrows. This combination of lesions produces the characteristic leonine facies of leprosy (Fig. 59).

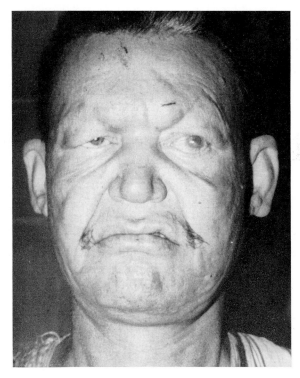

Fig. 59. Typical leonine facies of advanced lepromatous leprosy. The nodules are concentrated on ears, chin and malar and interciliary areas. eyebrow alopecia marked; palpebral palsy and corneal lepromata apparent.

Diffuse involvement of the mucous membranes of the nose, the mouth and the trachea is common, and respiratory occlusion has often been reported. There is almost always lepromatous infiltration in the reticuloendothelial cells of the liver, and amyloid deposition is usual in chronic cases. Renal failure secondary to amyloidosis is the most common cause of death in advanced lepromatous patients at the U.S. Public Health Service Leprosarium at Carville, Louisiana. Endocrine changes due to adrenal amyloidosis have also been noted. However, the most common endocrinopathy in lepromatous leprosy is infiltration of the testis with *M. leprae* and resultant testicular atrophy; gynaecomastia is a frequent sequel in male patients. Ocular involvement may occur in lepromatous as well as in tuberculoid leprosy, and it, too, may result in blindness. Infiltrates of lepra cells on the cornea and the iris produce partial or complete opacification. Uveitis is a common complication when a reaction occurs.

Diagnosis

The clinical diagnosis of leprosy is dependent on awareness of it as a possibility. Since there is no characteristic early skin lesion, leprosy should be included in the differential diagnosis of a wide variety of diseases involving the skin and the mucous membranes in those patients who have resided in one of the areas where leprosy is endemic. Anaesthesia is the cardinal sign and may precede any visible lesion. As pointed out in the section on pathology, other manifestations of leprosy vary with type of disease and the resistance of the host.

Confirmation of the diagnosis is by the detection of acid-fast *M. leprae*. These are sought in smears from incisions over nodules, the nasal mucous membranes, the face and the elbows and on skin and neural biopsies.

Serological and immunological techniques have not been very helpful in the diagnosis and classification of leprosy. False positive Wassermann reactions are common in lepromatous patients, but the *Treponema pallidum* immobilization test (TPI) will show negative results in the nonsyphilitic patient.

The lepromin (Mitsuda–Rost) reaction is a prognostic rather than a diagnostic test. An intradermal injection of a solution of *M. leprae* is used to assess the ability of the host to react to the organism. There is both an early (24-hour) and a delayed (4-week) reaction. If the reaction is positive, as judged by the size of the wheal and the nodule respectively, this is evidence of potential resistance to the infection. Positive results are found in almost all normal persons, in patients with tuberculoid leprosy, and in about 50 per cent of patients with mixed or dimorphous leprosy. A negative reaction implies low resistance and a poor prognosis. This is found in about 95 per cent of lepromatous patients and in about 50 per cent of those with the mixed variety. The test is obviously essential in advising contacts of leprous patients as to potential risk. It is also used in determining whether or not a person should be allowed to expose himself to contagious patients. An example of this function is in the hiring of leprosarium personnel. It is also used to judge response to therapy. It is of interest that BCG (bacillus Calmette–Guérin) vaccination will change a negative lepromin reaction to a positive one.

Treatment

BCG campaigns against tuberculosis have been followed by a sharp drop in the incidence of leprosy in endemic areas. The exact mechanism for the apparent effect of BCG in leprosy is not yet fully understood.

The sulphones have revolutionized the course and the prognosis of leprosy. The most important of this group is DDS (diaminodiphenyl sulphone). Substituted sulphones are broken down to this compound if given orally, and parenteral administration offers no advantages. The recommended initial dosage of DDS is 25 mg once weekly for 2 weeks. It is then increased by 25 mg every other week until a maximum of 500 mg weekly in divided daily doses is attained. The dosage should be maintained indefinitely or, at least, until 3 years after arrest of the disease. Drug resistance has rarely been reported with sulphones, and the prognosis of early cases in which the patients are on current drug therapy is excellent. There are a wide variety of other compounds of comparable efficacy if toxic reactions to DDS should occur.

One of the feared complications of sulphone treatment is a lepra reaction, which may complicate either tuberculoid or lepromatous leprosy. Erythema nodosum occurs frequently during treatment of lepromatous leprosy, and potentially serious reactivations also occur in the tuberculoid and the dimorphous types. Erythema multiforme also has been noted. Injudicious sulphone dosage is the most common cause of the lepra reaction. It is most often seen either when too great an initial dose is administered or when the dosage is increased too rapidly. A generalized exacerbation of all manifestations is common. Complications may include severe uveitis and iridocyclitis, iritis, orchitis, painful panniculitis, paralysing peripheral neuritis, generalized oedema and blister formation with histological evidence of massive multiplication of lepra cells.

Needless to say, sulphone administration should be drastically reduced and may even have to be discontinued during a reaction; adrenal steroids will control most severe reactions. As with any other infection, however, steroids are a two-edged sword. While controlling the reaction, they also break down basic defences against the leprotic infection. Thus they should be used cautiously and for as brief a time as possible.

Sulphone therapy has also drastically altered the ancient social and legal stigmata of leprosy. Whereas complete community isolation has been the *sine qua non* of leprosy control for centuries—in fact, during the Middle Ages a burial service was read over a leper declaring him legally dead (*sis mortuus mundo*), although yet living—leprologists today advise hospitalization more for the sake of patient therapy than as control of a public health hazard.

In advanced leprosaria there are well-trained ancillary staffs of nurses, social workers, chaplains, psychologists and occupational and physical therapists to help patients adjust both mentally and physically to the disease. Corrective surgical procedures and/or rehabilitation facilities now offer the hope of new function to damaged limbs. Plastic surgery is a helpful adjunct for those with lepromatous involvement of the face.

BIBLIOGRAPHY

Cochrane, R. G., and Davey, T. H. *Leprosy in Theory and Practice.* Baltimore, Williams and Wilkins Company, 1964.
International Journal of Leprosy: all volumes.
Rees, R., and Weddell, A. Transmission of Human Leprosy to the Mouse and its Clinical Implications. *Trans. R. Soc. trop. Med. Hyg.* **64,** 31, 1970.

17   Cholera

A disease that begins where other diseases end, with Death.

MAGENDIE

The cholera pandemics that scourged the world in the first half of the nineteenth century began in the Bengali basin and spread as far and as rapidly as man was then able to travel. The necessity for and the speed of travel in this age of interdependence have eliminated any possibility of localizing the disease. This was proved in the Egyptian outbreak of 1947, when 33,000 cases were reported within 3 months, and 2 out of 3 victims died. The seventh cholera pandemic began in Indonesia in 1961 and spread in the mid sixties throughout the Far and Middle East. In the last year of that decade cases appeared in Russia and fulminating outbreaks exploded for the first time in modern history throughout Africa. Localized epidemics were then noted in the Mediterranean littoral and in Southern Europe.

Until cholera can be eradicated at its Asiatic origins, the threat of infection at home or abroad will remain. Although the clinician in temperate climates will rarely have to manage a case, he will certainly be called on to advise or reassure the growing number of tourists, soldiers, migrants and businessmen exposed to the disease.

Pathological features

The havoc wreaked in its victims by cholera is frequently more evident to the clinical pathologist than to the histologist. Haematological, biochemical, immunological and bacteriological measurements are usually grossly deranged, whereas alterations in morbid anatomy may be minimal. The aetiological agent is a motile, gram-negative bacillus, shaped like a comma (*Vibrio comma* or *cholerae*), with a single polar flagellum. Several related vibrio strains (nonagglutinating or N.A.G. strains) have been isolated occasionally in choleraic stools but may be differentiated from the pathogenic *V. cholerae* by immunological techniques. The bacterium causing cholera is agglutinated by O group I type serum. Alternative methods of identification which utilize the antigen–antibody principle include complement fixation and visualization of bacteriolysis *in vivo*—the Pfeiffer phenomenon. Fermentation and haemolysin reactions are the bases for definitive identification and separation of the true *V. cholerae* from the mildly pathogenic El Tor strain.

Active human infections are essential for the inception and the maintenance of a cholera epidemic. Chronic human carriers or animal reservoirs do not exist. Transmission is via the anal–oral route and most frequently follows the ingestion of water or food contaminated with cholera stools or the handling, by unhygienic persons, of the sheets and the clothing of choleraic victims. Since the bacterium is destroyed in an acid medium, ingestion of a large quantity of water facilitates its survival by diluting gastric acidity. Multiplication of the vibrio appears to be most rapid in achlorhydric patients, and low or absent gastric acidity has been found in over 70 per cent of those with clinical cholera.

The organism multiplies in the alkaline small intestine, producing copious liquid excreta. There are almost as many theories to explain the source as there are litres of 'rice water' stools in a typical cholera case. There have been supporters for exudation from a damaged intestinal mucosa as the main cause, but regrettably there was no histological evidence to substantiate this view. Others backed the belief that a substance inhibited the reabsorption of fluid by altering the cellular sodium-pump mechanism, but there is inadequate evidence for this view. Nor do experimental observations support transudation as a significant mechanism in cholera. Increased intestinal secretion accounts for the majority of the isotonic cholera fluid production.

The stools have no faecal quality and lack protein, the albumin secretion of the small intestine being almost entirely reabsorbed in the colon. The total volume of excreta may exceed 50 l in 2 to 3 days. Continuous vomiting compounds the electrolyte imbalance (Table 9).

Table 9.   Changes in laboratory findings in severe cholera

Blood finding	In cholera patients	In normal persons
Sodium (meq/l)	125	140
Potassium (meq/l)	1·9 to 3·5	3·5 to 5·0
Chloride (meq/l)	115	102
Carbon dioxide (meq/l)	15	28
pH	7·28	7·40
Specific gravity	1·074	1·054

Haemoconcentration, with prolongation of the circulation time, and oliguria inactivate the normal respiratory and renal compensatory mechanisms. During the terminal uraemic phase, phosphate and sulphate retention accentuate the acidosis.

The gross and the microscopic tissue alterations in the choleraic victim during the uraemic phase are nonspecific. As in uraemia from any cause, vascular congestion and oedema are prominent in bowel, brain, heart and lungs. The kidneys, however, present a characteristic pattern of gross cortical necrosis, with no involvement of the medullary tubules.

The cholera victim who dies in collapse following voluminous rice-water stools bears the scars of local toxin damage and generalized dehydration. Scattered areas of surface haemorrhage interspersed with foci of lymphoid hyperplasia cover the mucosal surface of the small bowel. Peyer's patches in the terminal ileum are visibly hypertrophied. On histological section the villi are seen to be flattened and denuded of their epithelium, while the entire mucosa and submucosa are infiltrated with neutrophils and lymphocytes. There is rapid degeneration of intestinal pathological changes, and a necropsy, to be valid, must be done within 6 hours post mortem. Lymphoid proliferation is also evident in the thymus, the spleen and the mesenteric nodes.

The renal cortex is pale, with patchy areas of advanced ischaemia, while the medulla is congested. The adrenals appear normal on the usual macroscopic and microscopic examination, but lipoidophilic stains reveal a marked depletion in cortical cholesterol and ketosteroids. The remaining tissues and organs of the body show the effects of marked interstitial fluid loss and intravascular haemoconcentration. They are uniformly dry, pale and shrunken, with distended vascular channels full of thick, dark blood and multiple foci of petechial haemorrhage.

Clinical features

The majority of patients infected with *V. cholera* are asymptomatic or have signs and symptoms of a mild enteritis. The small percentage that develop classical cholera, however, present a clinical picture that is unforgettable. Although the course of cholera is traditionally divided into 5 stages, there is rarely any clear demarcation between them. The initial indication of infection is usually the sudden, explosive onset of copious diarrhoea in a previously healthy person. Since the incubation period lasts from 1 to 3 days, the physician in the temperate zone may see the first features of the disease in recent air travellers. During the first phase the patient is usually completely asymptomatic but may notice mild premonitory diarrhoea and vague malaise.

The stage of evacuation begins suddenly with voluminous, foul bowel movements, which soon become free of faeces and attain the characteristic rice-water colour. The evacuation may continue almost unabated for from 2 to 12 hours, with the fluid excreted exceeding 10 l. Vomiting may be constant, but there is usually neither nausea nor retching. As dehydration and electrolyte imbalance become more severe, excruciating muscular cramps and spastic rigidity are prominent. Tenesmus rarely occurs.

Profound shock ensues in the majority of cases, and the patient in the stage of collapse presents the moribund picture noted by Magendie. The skin is moist and cold, with cyanosis of the nails and the lips. There is a generalized shrinking and wrinkling of the dehydrated skin, most pronounced on the fingers and the face. The characteristic appearance of the hand has been referred to as 'washerwoman's fingers', while the sunken, dark-rimmed orbital cavities, the upturned eyes and the pinched nose make up the classic Hippocratic facies (Fig. 60). The patient is dyspnoeic and hypotensive, with an impalpable arterial pulse. Vomiting and diarrhoea abate, but oliguria or total anuria often develops.

Collapse may persist for from several hours to several days, and those who survive enter the stage of reaction, characterized by a recovery of formed stool, urinary flow, pulse, blood pressure and skin turgor and colour. The patient may develop the pattern of pyrexia with flushing of the skin and delirium referred to as cholera typhoid. During this phase pulmonary oedema and pneumonitis are frequent and often fatal complications if untreated. However, the majority of patients recover uneventfully within from 4 to 5 days.

About 10 per cent of untreated patients redevelop oliguria and anuria for a reason as yet unknown. The stage of uremia may be the end-result

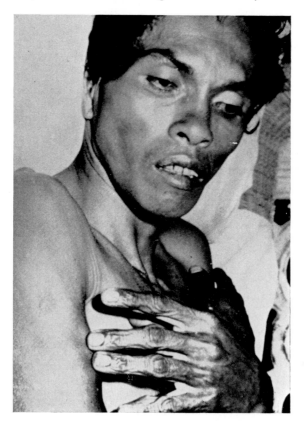

Fig. 60.   Man showing effects of cholera.

of the severe renal cortical damage which was described in the section on pathological features.

Diagnosis

The full-blown clinical picture of cholera coupled with a history of exposure can be confused with few other diseases. The absence of nausea, abdominal pain, tenesmus and retching easily differentiates it from the dysenteries or food poisoning. However, confirmation of the diagnosis by identification of the *V. cholerae* not only is desirable for the clinician but also is essential for the public health officer.

The organism may be seen by direct microscopy of the rice-water stools or the vomitus. Since the *V. cholerae* is about half the size ($1 \cdot 5$ to 2 microns) of the tubercle bacillus, oil immersion on the lens is necessary. The characteristic darting movements of the bacterium are seen most clearly in hanging-drop preparations on dark-field examination. The head-to-tail connections of a chain of vibrios may occasionally produce the distinctive fish-in-stream appearance of S-shaped curves. The vibrio is gram-negative; carbolfuchsin dye illuminates the characteristic comma shape with a terminal flagellum. Cultures positive for *V. cholerae* may be obtained within 8 hours, using an aerobic 1 per cent peptone medium at alkaline pH (optimal, $8 \cdot 5$). *V. cholerae* may be found in the stools of asymptomatic contact carriers for as long as 42 days after an attack. Definitive identification of the organism requires agglutination with O group I antisera. A rising titre of O agglutinins in the patient's serum provides alternative evidence of choleraic infection and is a technique especially useful for retrospective diagnosis after the stool is vibrio-free.

Treatment

Intravenous replacement of body fluids and electrolytes is the only effective therapy available. Rogers' regimen of hypertonic saline and bicarbonate stood unchallenged for over half a century. Lately investigators in both Calcutta and Formosa have found isotonic fluid replacement to be superior. The quantities administered are determined by careful, sequential clinical observations on the patient, particularly noting the radial pulse and skin turgor. Although following the blood specific gravity has been a traditional bedside test to estimate fluid needs in cholera patients, it is often an impossible task in epidemic settings and, more importantly, is not really more accurate than the astute clinical impression. The *average* patient with classical cholera will require from 20 to 25 litres of fluid replacement in the first 4 days.

Several litres of fluid should be infused in the initial hours, with a continuous but slower drip to follow. Because of the rapidity of electrolyte loss and the frequent anuria, blood pH and carbon dioxide content provide more valid measurements of choleraic acidosis than do urinary tests. Electrolyte deficits should be replaced via the infusion rather than by mouth.

Pressor agents may be required if hypotension is not corrected sufficiently by fluid replacement. Tetracycline shortens the clinical course of cholera. Using an isotonic fluid programme with added tetracycline, the Calcutta group has reduced the mortality of adequately treated cholera patients to less than I per cent. Attempts to develop an oral electrolyte solution for use in cholera are being studied.

Prevention

A cholera vaccine is available, and visitors to areas where cholera is endemic should be fully immunized at least 10 days before expected exposure. The protection elicited is neither uniform nor complete. Two subcutaneous injections (0·5 ml and I ml) a week apart are recommended, and the maximum antibody titre can be expected about 10 days after the second injection. Immunity is short-lived, and a booster dose every 4 to 5 months is advised. One of the main reasons to inoculate travellers going to endemic areas is to avoid the almost inevitable imposition of a locally prepared vaccine or—even worse—detention at a strange airport. Impure drinking water should, of course, be avoided. In the event of a clinical case being detected, local health and quarantine authorities should be notified at once. Strict isolation should be enforced, with sterilization of all linens, bed-pans and other utensils, and disposal of excreta only after chemical decontamination.

BIBLIOGRAPHY

Cahill, K. (ed.).   Cholera—A Symposium.   Bull. N.Y. Acad. Med. **47,** 1137–1212, 1971.
Felsenfeld, O.   The Cholera Problem.   St. Louis, Warren H. Green, Inc., 1967.
Wallace, C. K.   Cholera: A Continuing Threat and Challenge.   Int. Rev. trop. Med. **3,** 159, 1969.
De, S.   Cholera: Its Pathology and Pathogenesis.   Edinburgh, Oliver & Boyd, 1960.

18   Plague and Bartonellosis

Two 'exotic' bacterial diseases of the tropics occasionally present in temperate climates. Plague has captured the imagination of writers and artists for centuries and one of the best clinical and epidemiological descriptions is in Camus' classic novel, *La Peste*, detailing the impact of the disease on the city and population of Oran, Algeria. Bartonellosis is also one of those bizarre bacterial infections that have a fascinating history and an almost disproportionate impact on medical research.

PLAGUE

Although the clinical course of plague is as fulminating today as when pandemics of the disease decimated the world, it is more a potential than an actual health hazard. Fewer than 1,500 cases are reported annually to the WHO, the majority from endemic foci in northern Peru and central India. However, because it is an extremely wide-spread enzootic disease, plague is poised constantly on a delicate balance, and, when man and domestic rats contact the wild rodent reservoirs, human infection occurs (Fig. 61).

Rodent fleas, of which the most important is *Xenopsylla cheopis*, ingest *Pasteurella pestis* from infected rats. The organisms multiply in the oesophagus, or proventriculus, of the flea to such an extent that they cause blockage or impaction. As the thirsty flea sucks a second blood meal, it regurgitates bacilli into the wound site. Although wild rodents tolerate infection well and therefore are excellent reservoirs, domestic rats react in much the same way as man does. When they die, their fleas seek another source of food and man enters the infective cycle.

Sporadic cases that illustrate this epidemiological cycle are reported —for example, in the Southwestern United States—and devastating epidemics still occur in areas where man cohabitates closely with

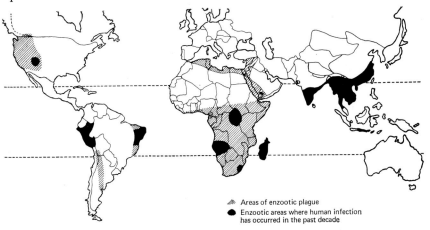

⫽ Areas of enzootic plague
● Enzootic areas where human infection has occurred in the past decade

Fig. 61.   World distribution of plague.

infected rats or when man-to-man transmission in pneumonic plague is not controlled.

P. pestis, the causative organism of plague, is a gram-negative, non-motile coccobacillus which is found in the sputum of pneumonic victims and in enlarged lymph nodes, or buboes, the spleen and the heart of bubonic plague patients. The virulence of *P. pestis* depends on the presence of somatic (V or W) antigens and a protective, surface antigen (F-I) and the production of a necrotizing endotoxin. The bacilli multiply in lymph nodes and disseminate only after toxic damage to neighbouring vascular beds has permitted spread via the bloodstream. Diffuse haemorrhage is common in epicardium, pericardium, spleen, liver, kidney, and brain. In victims of pneumonic plague, pulmonary and pleural haemorrhages are prominent.

The incubation period of human plague averages 3 to 5 days, but symptoms may be seen in primary pneumonic patients within 24 hours after infection. In all types the onset is acute, with fever, chills, confusion and prostration. In the pneumonic form of the disease cyanosis and coma are common; in bubonic plague painful, tender—and, occasionally, ulcerating—inguinal and cervical adenopathy is characteristic. In overwhelming septicaemic plague the victim may die before any signs are evident.

During an epidemic the presence of dying rats and contact cases makes confident clinical diagnosis possible. Laboratory confirmation in sporadic cases is essential. The organism can be visualized in gram or methylene blue preparations from buboes, sputum or blood in the living and from autopsy material of man, fleas or rodents. Culture on selective media enhances isolation. Thermoprecipitin and fluorescent antibody tests are also available.

Treatment in all types of plague is effective if it is given early in the disease; plague is usually fatal if therapy is delayed. Combinations of sulphamerazine in a daily dosage of 3 g for 1 week, streptomycin and tetracyclines together with serum antitoxin are recommended. The temperate-climate physician's concern with plague will be limited largely to advice for travellers in regard to prophylaxis. Both a living and a dead vaccine are available; they produce marked side-effects, they are only partially effective and they protect for less than 6 months. Only those persons who expect to be in contact with patients who are known to be infected or with infected animals should be advised to undergo inoculation. No nation currently requires plague vaccination for visitors. If contact is expected, prophylactic use of sulphonamides and streptomycin is advisable.

BARTONELLOSIS

Along the steep valley slopes of Peru, Colombia and Ecuador, bartonellosis is endemic. This bizarre and truly exotic disease is found only in humans and only within well-delineated limits of climate and altitude; it may present as a rapidly fatal, febrile anaemia, as a chronic dermatological disease, or as both.

The aetiological organism, *Bartonella bacilliformis*, is transmitted to man by the bite of an infective *Phlebotomus* sandfly. After an incubation period varying from 3 weeks to 4 months, acute symptoms may appear; most prominent are generalized pains in muscles and joints, tender enlargement of lymph nodes, fever and a sudden, severe macrocytic anaemia. This phase of bartonellosis is called Oroya fever or Carrión's disease (named after the young medical student who died of the infection while studying it). It usually lasts for 1 to 2 months; it can be diagnosed by visualization of *B. bacilliformis* within peripheral red blood cells, and, if untreated, it has a fatality rate exceeding 40 per cent.

Penicillin, streptomycin and the broad-spectrum antibiotics are highly effective in controlling the acute infection. The mode of action of these drugs is unknown; their impact appears to be primarily on concurrent secondary bacterial infections.

If the patient survives Oroya fever, a generalized haemangiomatous dermal eruption, verruga peruana, will be noted some 6 weeks later. Patients may develop verruga peruana as an initial manifestation of bartonellosis or, often, after asymptomatic Oroya fever. A verruga is formed by proliferating endothelial cells and newly formed capillaries. These eruptions may be miliary, nodular or ulcerative and lesions may persist for several years. Though there is no known treatment for verruga peruana, the prognosis is good, and one attack will provide a lasting immunity.

BIBLIOGRAPHY

Letgers, L., *et al.*   Clinical and Epidemiological Notes on a Defined Outbreak of Plague in Vietnam.   *Am. J. trop. Med. Hyg.* **19,** 639, 1970.
WHO Expert Committee on Plague.   Fourth Report, Tech. Rep. Ser. No. 447.   Geneva, 1971.
Schultz, M.   A History of Bartonellosis (Carrión's Disease).   *Am. J. trop. Med. Hyg.* **17,** 503, 1968.

145

IV VIRAL DISEASES

---

19 Smallpox

The discovery in 1798 of a simple, safe and successful vaccination for the prevention of smallpox provided the means for eliminating a disease that has scourged mankind from its earliest days. Yet a century and a half passed before a world-wide eradication scheme was begun, and only in recent years has the annual incidence of over 100,000 cases been, almost unbelievably, reduced to a few hundred. By applying all the modern methods for disease control a World Health Organization smallpox campaign succeeded in inoculating 100 million Africans within 3 years and virtually eliminating this disease from that continent.

Smallpox exemplified the potential threat of tropical diseases in temperate climates. It is highly contagious; it is often fatal, and its survivors are sorely disfigured. During the silent, 12-day incubation period an infected person from an area where the physician's index of suspicion makes diagnosis easy can travel by airplane to cities and towns where the abrupt, febrile onset may be mistaken for influenza and the rash may be mistaken for chickenpox. The outcome is even more confusing and tragic when the patient possesses a 'valid' vaccination certificate signed unwittingly before the winter cruise or business trip by a 'helpful' physician neighbour.

Because smallpox is rare, community protection by vaccination is often low, and rapid transmission must be expected if early diagnosis, isolation and other precautionary measures are not enforced.

Pathological features
The virus causing classical smallpox, or variola major, is morphologically identical with the virus of variola minor, or alastrim, and with the virus of vaccinia or cowpox, It can be grown on chick chorioallantoic membranes and tissue culture and can be demonstrated indirectly by complement-fixation, haemagglutination and gel-diffusion

precipitation techniques. Intracytoplasmic inclusions (Guarnieri bodies) and elementary virus particles (Paschen bodies) can be found on biopsy and in smears from skin and mucous membrane lesions. The virus is resistant to drying and may remain infective for long periods in contaminated bedding and dust.

The portal of entry for man is usually the upper respiratory tract, with direct inoculation as an alternative means. During the noninfective incubation period the pox viruses develop in respiratory lymphoid tissue. Haematogenous dissemination occurs at this time, and virus proliferation continues in the epidermis, where sharply localized foci of epithelial cells undergo characteristic reticulating degeneration. Similar degenerative changes occur in mucous membranes. Rupture of these swollen cells results in surface vesiculation and 'balloon' degeneration of the basal layers (Fig. 62). Pustulation occurs even in the absence of secondary bacterial invasion, but superimposed streptococcal infection is the rule rather than the exception. The severity of permanent pitting on the face is related to the extent of retraction and granulation of damaged sebaceous glands, while scar formation on the body is usually caused by damage from secondary infection. Other pathological changes include diffuse bronchopneumonia, hepatosplenomegaly with local infarction and capsulitis, renal cortical necrosis and widespread petechial haemorrhages in the heart, the intestine, the kidney, the liver, the spleen, the eyes and the skin.

Clinical features

In smallpox, as in all diseases, there can be a variety of clinical façades. Depending on host resistance, the virulence of the infecting dose and the degree of immunity, the same virus can cause a fulminating, haemorrhagic death or a subclinical infection without a rash. After the incubation period of 12 days there is an abrupt onset of chills, fever to 104°F, severe backache, nausea, vomiting and prostration. A dusky, erythematous or petechial rash, most marked in the inguinal region— the so-called bathing trunks pattern—may or may not be present. This period of toxaemic viraemia lasts for from 3 to 4 days and is followed by a feeling of relative well-being and the eruption of the focal rash by which the disease has been recognized since antiquity.

The skin lesions are delicate macules often found initially on the tip of the nose, the forehead and the lateral aspects of the neck. Within 2 days the macules evolve into shotlike papules and, after another 2 days, into vesicles. The vesicles become umbilicated and pustular, with scab formation beginning approximately 9 days from the onset of the rash

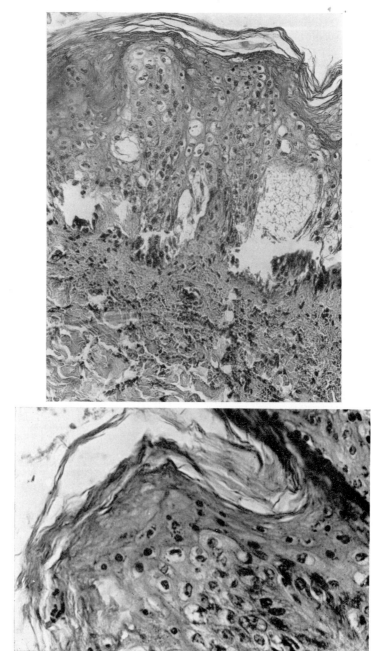

Fig. 62. Biopsy specimen of smallpox lesion. *Top*, unilocular vesiculation; *bottom*, several intracytoplasmic Guarnieri bodies.

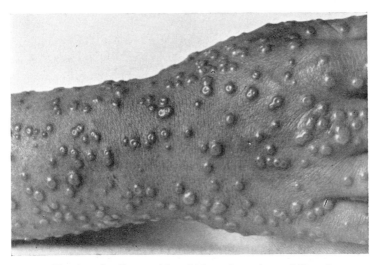

Fig. 63.   Smallpox vesicles which are becoming umbilicated.

(Fig. 63). In lesions uncomplicated by secondary infection, the crusts usually have separated within 3 weeks.

This knowledge of the natural history of smallpox will permit the clinician to resolve his most common and serious concern with the disease: its differentiation from varicella or chickenpox. Although the lesions of severe varicella can mimic superficially those of mild variola, a careful history and examination will almost always indicate the correct diagnosis (Table 10).

Table 10.   Distinguishing features for bedside diagnosis of variola and varicella

Features of disease	Smallpox	Chickenpox
Onset	Sudden	Gradual
Fever	Falls with appearance of rash	Persists during rash
Rash		
Distribution	Centrifugal	Centripetal
Age	Uniform	Varied; appears in crops
Vesicles	Shotty; umbilicated	Soft
Histology	Multilocular; intracytoplasmic Guarnieri bodies	Unilocular; intranuclear Lipschütz bodies
White blood cell count per cubic millimetre	15,000 to 20,000	3,000 to 5,000

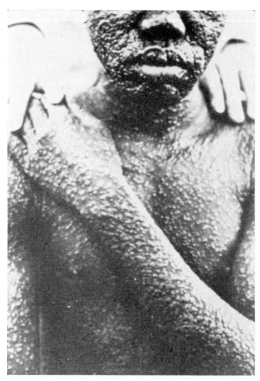

Fig. 64. Characteristic distribution of smallpox lesions, with greater concentration on the face and the extremities than on the torso.

A vaccination scar in a child or the history of a recent, successful smallpox inoculation in an adult provides the best evidence against smallpox. However, when these are lacking and the clinical picture or history of exposure is at all suggestive, the illness should be considered as smallpox until evolution of the infection, laboratory evidence or expert opinion rules otherwise. Public health authorities should be notified at once and proper preventive measures initiated. It is far better to err temporarily in this way than to allow a patient with highly contagious smallpox to pose a risk to the community while a final diagnosis is being debated.

Diagnosis

The presence of smallpox virus can be confirmed by serological, culture or histological techniques; and details should be sought in specialized virology or laboratory texts.

Treatment

There is no specific treatment for smallpox. Scrupulous nursing care, proper fluid balance and use of early vaccination and V.I.G. (vaccinia-immune globulin, a gamma globulin suspension prepared from recently vaccinated individuals) may modify the disease. Antibiotics have been reported to lower the incidence of septic dermatitis and broncho-pneumonia, but adequate, controlled studies have not been done in this area. N-methylisatin b-thiosemicarbazone has antivaccinal activity *in vitro* and has been successful both as a therapeutic and as a prophylactic agent. Steroids may be of use in the fulminating, malignant type of smallpox, but again no controlled data are available.

Jennerian vaccination is the most important measure in the prevention of smallpox, the control of epidemics and the treatment of patients with recent exposure. A successful vaccination performed within 3 days after exposure to an infective patient often elicits an antibody response sufficient to prevent clinical manifestations of the disease.

Properly administered, smallpox vaccination is one of the safest tools in the medical armamentarium. However, there are rare complications,

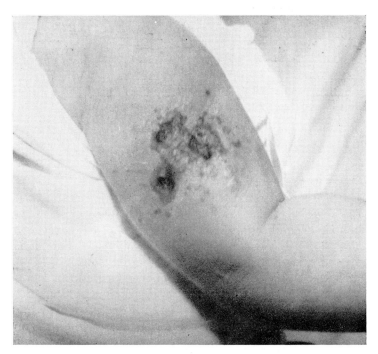

Fig. 65.   Localized vaccinia gangrenosa in an Egyptian infant.

which include encephalopathy, myocarditis and autogenous or accidental spread from scratching of the vaccination site and transfer of the infection to the eye, the buccal mucosa and other sites. Generalized vaccinial eruption very rarely occurs between the sixth and the ninth days in an otherwise normal primary vaccination. The incidence of this complication and of gangrenous vaccinia is enormously increased if the patient has eczema (Fig. 65) or any open skin lesion. Vaccination is contraindicated in pregnant women, except when risk from known exposure is certain, in those with chronic diseases such as diabetes, or during debilitated phases of tuberculosis, the leukaemias and the hypogammaglobulinaemias. V.I.G. should be administered prophylactically with vaccination in these instances.

BIBLIOGRAPHY

Dixon, C. *Smallpox.* London, Churchill, 1962.
Marsden, J. P. On the Diagnosis of Smallpox. *Brit. J. clin. Pract.* **16** (suppl. 1–9), 1962.
Hopkins, D., *et al.* Smallpox in Sierra Leone: The 1968–69 Eradication Program. *Am. J. trop. Med. Hyg.* **20**, 697, 1971.

20   Yellow Fever and Arbor Virus Infections

YELLOW FEVER

There are few more exciting chapters in the history of medicine than that of yellow fever. The devastation that followed epidemics caused panic in ports around the world, and the spread of yellow fever through colonial and nineteenth century America left a lasting imprint on international quarantine and local health rules. Outbreaks not only forced political and economic changes, and polarized the contagionist versus the anticontagionist groups in the development of public health, but had a profound impact on the scientific approach to infectious diseases. Noble men gave their lives in self-experimentation searching for the truth of yellow fever. Until the 'yellow jack' was conquered, construction of the Panama Canal was not feasible, and American ports were exposed to fulminating periodic outbreaks. In 1878 there were 13,000 deaths from yellow fever in Mississippi River towns, and as late as 1905 some 5,000 cases were reported from New Orleans.

Although yellow fever has largely faded from view in the last half century in temperate climates, it remains an explosive threat. Outbreaks in Ethiopia and Senegal in the sixties afflicted several hundred thousand persons. The recognition that 'jungle' or rural yellow fever is maintained as a zoonosis among forest monkeys eliminated any hope that the disease could be totally eradicated. Jungle yellow fever is transmitted by several species of *Haemagogus* mosquitoes in the Americas and by *Aedes africanus* and *A. simpsoni* in Africa. Man is only accidentally infected either by canopy-dwelling mosquitoes that are brought to ground level when trees are felled or by monkeys coming down to forage in gardens on the forest edge. Once infected, however, man can serve as a reservoir for the urban *A. aegypti*, and human epidemics can be initiated (Fig. 66, 67).

The jungle variety of the disease has moved progressively northward from Panama in recent decades and monkeys in southern Mexico are now infected. Since vector eradication programmes either have failed or have been discontinued, the entire eastern seaboard of the United States remains a receptive area for the reintroduction and the

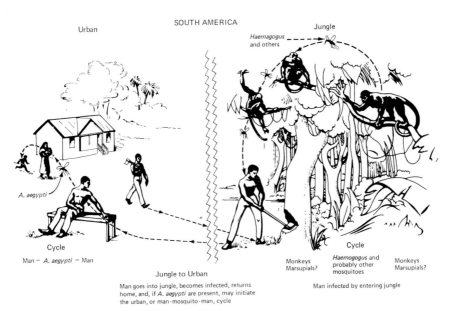

Fig. 66. Epidemiology of sylvan yellow fever: South America.

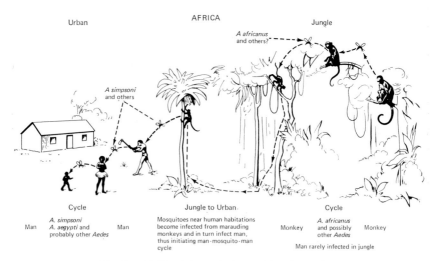

Fig. 67.   Epidemiology of sylvan yellow fever: Africa.

spread of yellow fever. The reality of this threat for the Americas was proved recently by a small epidemic of yellow fever in Trinidad, after the island had been free from the disease for thirty-odd years.

Table 11.   Some tropical arbor viruses causing significant human disease

Group	Virus	Type of disease	Distribution
A	Chikungunya	Denguelike	East Africa
	Onyong-nyong	Denguelike	Uganda
	Venezuelan encephalitis	Encephalitis	Venezuela, Colombia, Brazil
	Yellow fever	(See text)	Africa, South and Central America
B	Dengue Type 1	(See text)	Central America, Asia
	Dengue Types 2–6	Haemorrhagic fever	Far East
	Uganda S	Denguelike	East Africa
	West Nile	Denguelike	North Africa, Middle East
	Murray Valley	Encephalitis	New Guinea, Australia
	Kyasanur Forest	Haemorrhagic fever	India
	Japanese B	Encephalitis	Asia
Ungrouped			
	Sandfly fever	Denguelike	Italy, Egypt
	Rift Valley	Denguelike	East and West Africa
	Argentinian haemorrhagic fever	Haemorrhagic fever	South America

Pathological features

The virus of yellow fever is a member of the immunologically related Group B arbor (arthropod-borne) viruses, and infection with any one of these (Table 11) elicits antibodies which are protective, to a degree, against the whole group. Infection with yellow fever produces a permanent immunity, and there has never been a well-documented clinical case of reinfection. There are many strains of the yellow fever virus. For many years the South American variant was thought to produce a disease unrelated to the African virus. The major laboratory strains, distinguished by the organ primarily involved, are the hepatotropic, or viscerotropic, and the neurotropic, with varying degrees of virulence allowing further subdivisions. The 17-D strain of the viscerotropic group and the neurotropic Dakar strain have been used most widely in the preparing of yellow fever vaccines. Although these virus strains primarily attack different organs, both multiply in the liver. Inoculation with one interferes with the pathogenicity of the other.

The anatomic changes of yellow fever were long confused by Noguchi's belief that *Leptospira* was the aetiological agent and by the hepatitis that so often accompanied inoculation experiments when the virus was suspended in human serum. Histological changes in the liver

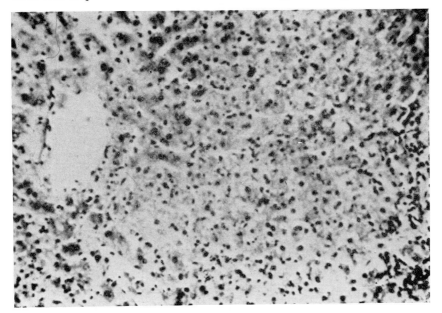

Fig. 68. Postmortem liver section from an African man demonstrating marked midzonal necrosis characteristic of yellow fever.

in the advanced case of yellow fever include midzonal necrosis, acido-
philic coagulum in the cytoplasm of parenchymal cells (Councilman
bodies), occasional intranuclear inclusions and a striking absence of
inflammatory cells (Fig. 68). In the milder cases, there may be focal
fatty infiltration and dilatation of the sinusoids, without necrosis. In
severe cases the kidneys are swollen and icteric, with degenerative
changes which are most pronounced in the proximal convoluted tubules.
Fatty infiltration with degeneration is also prominent in the myo-
cardium and the conducting system. In human yellow fever, cerebral
involvement is minimal and nonspecific. Perivascular haemorrhage
in the brain occurs, but it is merely part of a general haemorrhagic
diathesis which is most pronounced in the skin and in the mucous
membranes of the stomach and the intestinal tract.

Clinical features

Since the incubation period of yellow fever varies from 3 to 6 days,
it is possible for an air traveller from a zone where the disease is endemic to develop the initial symptoms in a temperate climate. The
majority of patients with the disease have only minor symptoms, and
only a small percentage develop the classical clinical picture. However,
in this minority, a characteristic picture evolves. The onset is sudden,
with severe headache, backache, muscular pains, epistaxis, nausea,
haematemesis, melaena, icterus and marked albuminuria. The temperature may reach 105°F, but the pulse remains slow (Faget's sign).
Insomnia and irritability are prominent and may persist for 3 to 4
days. A brief period of remission usually occurs, during which the
patient feels much better, although pathological processes may be continuing unabated. Toxaemia then reappears, and all the manifestations
of the initial phase are accentuated. It is during this phase, which may
last for several weeks, that the patient may die from hepatic and renal
failure or from uncontrolled haemorrhages. Even during convalescence,
sudden deaths occur from myocardial failure and cardiac arrhythmias.

Diagnosis

Leukopenia is present during all phases of yellow fever except in
those cases in whom secondary bacterial invasion complicates convalescence. Anaemia will occur if haemorrhage is pronounced. Results
of liver function tests, including prothrombin estimations, are deranged.
The urine may contain over 5 g of albumin per day, and the blood urea
nitrogen is often markedly elevated.

Specific diagnosis can be accomplished in several ways. During the initial period of infection the virus can be isolated directly from the blood by inoculation into the brains of mice or into nonimmune Rhesus monkeys. After a suitable incubation period, neutralization studies on the monkey blood or the mouse brain suspensions are performed with hyperimmune serum from laboratory animals known to be infected with yellow fever. A more elaborate procedure is the mouse-protection test, in which a known quantity of yellow fever virus suspension is inoculated into mice with 'unknown' serum from a patient. If antibodies are present, the mouse will be protected. If the serum is non-immune, the mouse will die of a fatal encephalitis.

Serological methods are accurate and diagnostic if a rising antibody titre can be demonstrated. Antibodies against the yellow fever virus are produced very rapidly and may be present even during the late viraemic stage. A combination of the haemagglutination and complement-fixation tests is often employed. Technical details for performing and interpreting the tests are available in texts on virology or in the paper covering our studies in East Africa cited below. The main drawback to all serological methods for the diagnosis of yellow fever is cross-reaction with other Group B arbor viruses. Histological examination of liver sections after death may allow retrospective diagnosis by revealing typical midzonal fatty change.

Treatment

There is no specific treatment for yellow fever. Supportive measures, such as glucose infusions for alleviation of hepatic glycolysis, vitamin K injections for correction of bleeding tendencies and the maintenance of fluid balance in order to avoid complicating renal damage, are important. *A. aegypti* control remains essential for community protection. Vaccination is the key to personal prophylaxis. If the vaccine is properly administered, either by subcutaneous inoculation or, in mass programmes, by scarification, there are almost no failures in eliciting an antibody response. The antibody titre reaches a protective level within 8 to 10 days and remains at this level for at least 10 years.

Postvaccination reactions with the 17-D strain have been rare since concomitant human serum administration (now known to be a cause of serum hepatitis) was discontinued in 1943. A few cases of nonfatal encephalitis have been reported, but, among the many millions of vaccinations, the incidence of this complication is negligible. The Dakar neurotropic vaccine has been used very widely in Africa because it is inexpensive and easily administered; however, fatal encephalitis has

occurred in several such vaccination programmes. At the present time
it is recommended that a patient visiting Africa or Central or South
America undergo vaccination with the 17-D strain at least 10 days
before expected arrival in an area where yellow fever is endemic.
Infants under 1 year of age and pregnant women should be exempted
unless the risk is extremely high, since the incidence of encephalitis is
significantly greater in their case.

ARBOR VIRUS INFECTIONS

The antigenically related Group B arbor viruses produce diseases which
are less severe than yellow fever, although similar to it in many ways.
Inoculation of 17-D vaccine into experimental animals will ameliorate
the effects of a simultaneously injected dengue virus, and it has been
suggested that cross-protection is also evident in the epidemiology of
this group. Dengue is endemic in the Far East, where yellow fever does
not occur, and is modified or absent in African and American areas
infested with yellow fever. The recent outbreak of 30,000 cases of a
denguelike illness in the Caribbean proves that this pattern of distribution is far from absolute. However, the immunity induced by these
Group B viruses is not lasting, and reinfections do occur. All are transmitted by arthropods, with *A. aegypti* the most important tropical vector.
    Dengue, Uganda S and West Nile fevers are closely allied clinically
and immunologically. As in yellow fever, leukopenia is usually marked,
Faget's sign is often present, and the clinical pattern can be separated
into phases of infection, remission and increased toxaemia. They are
short-term (less than 10 days), acute febrile diseases causing severe
headache, muscle and joint pains ('breakbone fever'), a saddlebacked
temperature curve with peaks to 104°F on the second or third day of
the illness, with a lesser rise on the seventh day, and a transient,
rubellalike rash.
    Murray Valley, Kyasanur Forest and Japanese B encephalitides are
related Group B viruses which are endemic in parts of the tropics and,
occasionally, cause clinical epidemics in the temperate zones. On the
other hand, eastern and western equine encephalomyelitides are
examples of Group B viral diseases which are endemic in the United
States but are responsible also for fulminating outbreaks in tropical
America. There is no specific treatment for any of these diseases, and
medical assistance is limited to supportive measures. However, the
physician can reassure the patient during the periods of extreme pros-

tration that characterize dengue, Uganda S and West Nile fevers that recovery is almost always complete within 10 days.

Several Group A arbor viruses of the tropics, including those that cause Onyong-nyong fever in East Africa and Chikungunya fever in Tanzania, also are responsible for short-term febrile illnesses, with insignificant morbidity and mortality. On the other hand, Venezuelan encephalitis is a frequently fatal Group A arbor virus disease.

Among the ungrouped tropical arbor viruses causing disease in man, those of sandfly fever in Italy and Egypt and of Rift Valley fever in Africa produce denguelike illnesses, while that of Argentinian haemorrhagic fever has caused a sizable number of fatalities in South America, as well as in many temperate areas.

There is an ever-growing number of arbor virus infections recognized as significant illnesses of man. A registry of these is maintained by the American Committee on Arthropod-borne Viruses.

BIBLIOGRAPHY

Strode, G., *et al.*   *Yellow Fever.*   New York, McGraw–Hill, 710 pp., 1951.

Councilman, W.   Description of Pathological Histology of Yellow Fever.   *U.S. Marine Hospital Service Pub. Health Bull.* **2,** 151, 1890.

Henderson, B., Metselane, D., and Cahill, K.   Yellow Fever Immunity in Uganda, Kenya and Somalia.   *Bull. WHO* **38,** 229, 1968.

Taylor, R. *Catalogue of Arthropod-borne Viruses of the World.*   *P.H.S. Public. No.* 1760.   Washington, D.C., U.S. Gov't Printing Office, 1967.

21 Tropical Treponemal and Rickettsial Diseases

TROPICAL TREPONEMATOSES

It is thought that treponemal infections evolved in the primeval, moist jungles of Africa, altered in highland and arid desert communities, and finally halted in an arrested state in the Americas. Between the florid sores of yaws and the limited depigmentation of pinta lie a variety of lesions with a multitude of local names including bejel, sita, njovera, dichuchwa and radesyga. These diseases are of interest to the temperate-climate physician because of their endemicity, chronicity and curability, as well as for the light they cast on our own treponemal disease, syphilis. All treponemal infections are morphologically and serologically indistinguishable; none of the tropical variants are venereal diseases. Some authorities contend that all treponematoses are different manifestations of one disease (the Unitarian Theory of Hudson); nevertheless, clinical and epidemiological patterns permit the differentiation of yaws from bejel and other intermediate forms and from pinta.

Yaws. In common with all tropical treponematoses, yaws is a disease of squalor. It flourishes in the hot, humid lowlands of Africa, Asia and Central America, especially where nakedness is the custom, crowded conditions are common, and water is scarce. By conservative estimates, more than fifty million persons are infected with yaws. Though the causative organism, *Treponema pertenue*, is indistinguishable from *T. pallidum*, the natural history of the disease is markedly different from that of syphilis.

Transmission is nonvenereal, with direct contact as the major method of spread, and mechanical conveyance by the *Hippelates pallipes* fly as a minor means. The primary lesion is an inconspicuous papule which is found most frequently in children of from 2 to 5 years of age. The

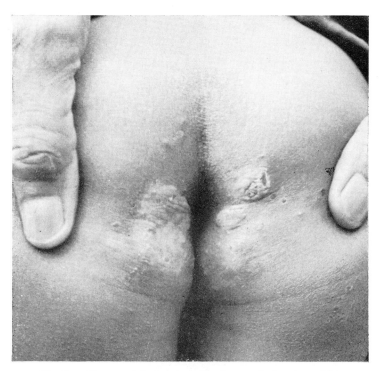

Fig. 69. Characteristic location of early yaws lesions in a child.

'mother' papule, which erupts 3 to 5 weeks after infection, is pruritic but painless, and it may enlarge into a hypertrophic papilloma 2 cm wide (Fig. 69). Papillomata often erupt over the body surface within a few weeks after the initial lesion, but they may not appear for years. The concept of latency is particularly important to the understanding of the course of yaws, for 'early' lesions can erupt long after the initial sore and several crops of early lesions may appear within the first 5 years of infection, each healing without evidence of scarring.

Secondary skin sores are more numerous and disfiguring. These 'daughter' or 'typical' yaws lesions are yellow, raised, wartlike or raspberrylike, and often have central ulcerations. Serpiginous and circinate papillomata, mucosal plaques and hyperkeratotic or ulcerating lesions of the palms and the soles are other varieties of early yaws. Once again, long latent periods may separate multiple secondary relapses, and healing is without scar formation.

Bone and joint lesions of early yaws also heal spontaneously without residual damage. Polydactylitis is characteristic of early yaws in children.

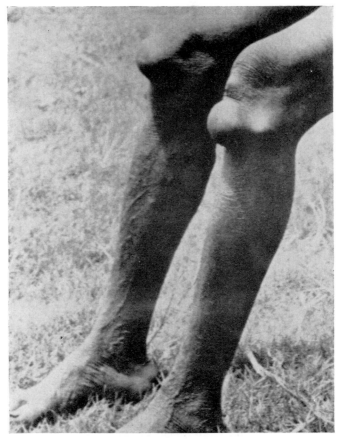

Fig. 70. Juxta-articular nodes of late yaws.

Periostitis is frequent, especially involving the radius, the ulna and the nasal maxilla; ganglions and transient hydroarthrosis may occur. The aetiological relationship of yaws to sabre tibia has not yet been proved.

Within 5 years of infection yaws becomes a destructive disease, and 'late' lesions of both skin and bones produce permanent damage (Figs. 70 and 71). Internal organs are not involved. Gummatous nodules with central ulceration may persist as indolent sores or resolve with residual scar and keloid formation. Marked hyperkeratosis of the palms and the soles may cause Dupuytren-like contractures. Gummatous periostitis and osteitis produce an X-ray picture of mixed translucency and density. Osteomyelitis, suppurative dactylitis and complete collapse of the nasal septum (gangosa) may complicate the course of late yaws.

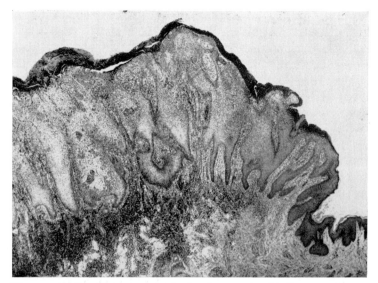

Fig. 71. Section of a yaws papule showing pseudoepitheliomatous hyperplasia, elongation and branching of rete pegs and necrosis of the superficial epidermis with marked mononuclear infiltration.

The diagnosis of yaws can be confirmed by visualization of *T. pertenue* in dark-field preparations or on Levaditi-stained smears obtained from ulcer edges. Immunological evidence provided by positive Kahn, Wasserman or T.P.I. tests is supportive but nonspecific, since treponemal infections cannot be differentiated in the serology laboratory. Partial cross-immunity appears to exist with syphilis; when yaws is eradicated, the incidence of venereal syphilis rises. Nonetheless, there have been many cases in which double infection with *T. pallidum* and *T. pertenue* has been demonstrated.

Penicillin cures yaws. Almost all early infections are healed after a course of 500,000 units daily for 7 days. Late cases usually respond to a regimen of 1 million units daily for 10 days. In mass programmes a single injection of 1·2 million units of long-acting penicillin has proved effective.

Intermediate forms. Yaws becomes less florid as the geography changes from moist lowland to dry savannah. Along the desert borders of Africa and the Middle East, bejel and other endemic syphilidides are the dominant nonvenereal treponemal infections. The onset of these diseases usually occurs later in childhood than does that of yaws. Lesions are concentrated on moist areas such as the mouth, the axilla, the inguinal area and the rectum. The frequency of sores on the buccal mucosal junctions has caused the common drinking cup to be incriminated as a mechanical means of spread. Late palmar lesions and bone destruction are common, but no organ damage occurs. Serological tests for syphilis are positive and, though visualization of treponema from wound aspirates is desirable, there is nothing pathognomonic in their morphology. Treatment with penicillin is curative.

Pinta. Throughout much of tropical America another nonvenereal treponemal infection flourishes. Pinta (so called from the Spanish word for 'spot') is a purely cutaneous disease caused by *T. carateum*. Primary lesions, observed only under experimental conditions, appear 10 to 16 days after artificial inoculation. The natural means of transmission is uncertain; direct contact is presumed to be the major method of spread, though vector transmission by both *Simulium* and *Hippelates* flies has been proved to be possible. The secondary lesions, or pintids, are scaly, squamous papules on an erythematous base. As the lesions become inactive, achromia becomes more prominent (Fig. 72). These areas of slaty depigmentation are usually bilateral and symmetric and are associated with concurrent desquamation, lichenization and hyperkeratosis. There is no latent period in pinta, and the tertiary lesions evolve from pintids. Treponemes can be found in juice expressed from

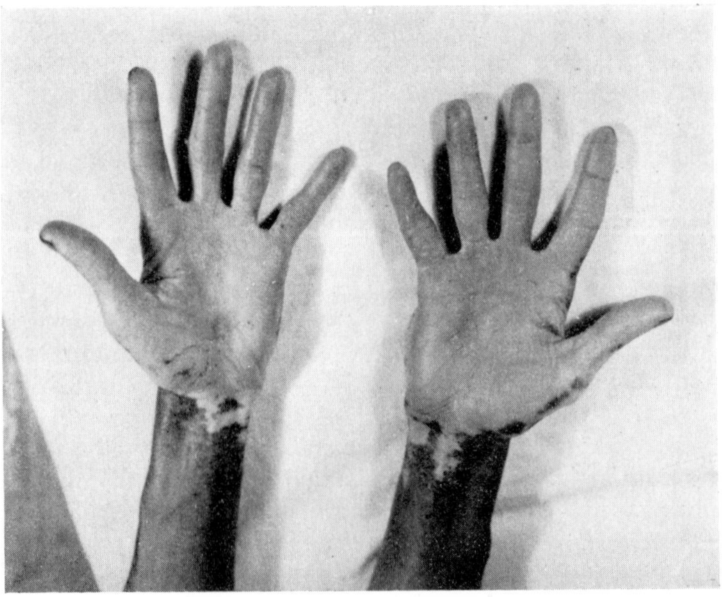

Fig. 72. Classical late pinta, showing total achromia of the palms with moderate hyperkeratosis.

scrapings of pintids but they are rare in the achromic, late lesions. Penicillin will cure pinta but will not reverse late depigmentary changes.

A far more important treponemal dermatosis is tropical phagedenic ulcer.

Tropical ulcer. Throughout undeveloped areas of Africa and Asia acute ulcers of the leg are common, disabling and disfiguring. The majority are categorized as 'tropical ulcer'. Though this term has often served as a wastebucket for nonspecific diagnoses, recent work permits the proper classification of many cases as *tropical phagedenic ulcer* (TPU). Although the aetiology of TPU remains uncertain, distinct clinical and laboratory patterns exist.

The lesion begins as a small papule on the lower leg of malnourished young adults and evolves within a few days into a painful, purulent ulcer 6 to 10 cm in diameter (Fig. 73). Tissue necrosis is extensive and the tibia is frequently exposed; the entire foreleg may slough in severe

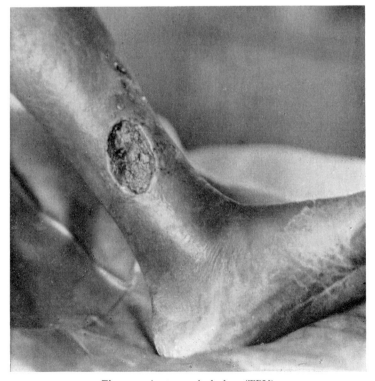

Fig. 73.   Acute tropical ulcer (TPU).

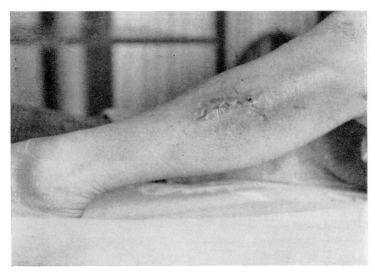

Fig. 74. Friable scar in a 'healed' TPU.

cases. However, most lesions evolve into a chronic ulcer with raised, firm edges; cicatrization may require months, and the scar is often fixed to deeper tissues and is incomplete and easily broken down (Fig. 74).

Scrapings from early ulcers contain *T. vincenti*, but the exact role of these organisms in the pathogenesis of TPU is uncertain. A wide range of bacterial contaminants can be isolated from chronic lesions. Differential diagnosis in the tropics includes diphtheria, yaws, cutaneous leishmaniasis, sickle-cell disease and dracunculosis as well as afflictions such as tuberculosis, syphilis, diabetes and varicose stasis which are found in temperate climates also. Acute TPU heals rapidly under local and systemic treatment with penicillin or aureomycin. Metronidazole (Flagyl) has recently been employed with success. Although no specific deficiency of vitamin or protein can be demonstrated, general nutritional supplements do enhance antibiotic therapy. Debridement of chronic ulcers and surgical excision with grafting may be necessary in late lesions.

TROPICAL RICKETTSIOSES

The majority of human rickettsial infections occur in the temperate zone. The most devastating example of this class of infections, epidemic typhus (*Rickettsia prowazeki*), is a disease of cold climates; even in endemic areas of the subtropics outbreaks are limited to the winter season and the highland regions. The Rocky Mountains of the United States provide the eponym for a whole group of rickettsial fevers (*R. rickettsii* etc.), and another of these, rickettsialpox (*R. akari*), is contracted only in New York City. However, in local areas of the tropics several types of typhus are significant health hazards; the most important are scrub typhus in the Far East and the boutonneuse tick typhus infections in North and Central Africa.

To provide the temperate-climate clinician with detailed descriptions of the rickettsioses would be similar to 'carrying coals to Newcastle' (Table 12). A few generalized comments will permit adequate recollection of the pathogenesis of these diseases and also serve to stimulate

Table 12.   Differentiating features of the human rickettsioses

Disease	Parasite	Vector	Rash	Eschar and adenopathy	Weil–Felix
Epidemic typhus	*R. prowazeki*	Louse	Trunk	o	OX–19
Murine typhus	*R. mooseri*	Flea	Trunk	o	OX–19
Scrub typhus	*R. tsutsugamuchi*	Mite	Trunk	+	OX–K
Spotted fevers					
Rocky Mountain	*R. rickettsii*	Tick	Limbs	o	OX–19 and OX–2
African	*R. conorii*	Tick	Limbs	+	OX–19 and OX–2
Australian	*R. australis*	Tick	General	+	OX–19 and OX–2
New York	*R. akari*	Mite	Trunk	+	Negative
Trench fever	*R. quintana*	Louse	Trunk	o	Unknown
Q fever	*R. burnetti*	Tick	None	o	Negative

their inclusion in the differential diagnosis of illnesses that are characterized by fever and a rash.

Except for epidemic typhus (of which man is the only proved reservoir of infection) the human rickettsioses are zoonoses transmitted to man by arthropods. There may or may not be local and lymphatic evidence of the bite site. The endothelial linings of small blood vessels are most heavily parasitized, and thromboses with perivascular haemorrhage and polymorphonuclear infiltration comprise the basic pathological lesions. These, which are often termed Wolbach's nodules, may be found in all organs of the body but are most pronounced in the skin, the brain, the lungs and the heart. The clinical syndrome of sudden fever, prostration, delirium, diffuse neurological

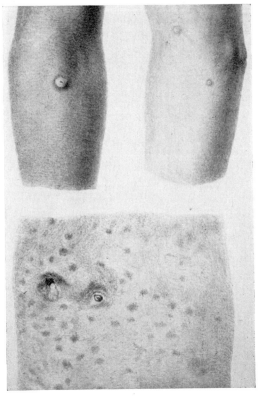

V

Fig. 75. Primary lesions and eruptions in a Japanese case of scrub typhus.

disturbances and a rash follows an incubation period of 10 days (average). Signs and symptoms persist for 2 weeks and then the fever, in favourable cases, falls by lysis. Complete convalescence often requires 6 months. Isolation of rickettsiae rarely is possible, and laboratory confirmation is based usually on serological tests. The Weil–Felix reaction (using 3 different *Proteus* strains as antigen) is a nonspecific but very useful test. Group- and type-specific complement-fixation and agglutination tests are even more valuable, but purified antigens are difficult to obtain. Treatment with chloramphenicol and other broad spectrum antibiotics is effective; the drugs are not rickettsiocidal and inadequate courses of therapy are associated with a high percentage of relapses. A vaccine prepared from strain E *R. prowazeki* is available for immunization. The indications for and the value of its use are discussed in Chapter 24.

BIBLIOGRAPHY

Hackett, C.   On the Origin of the Human Treponematoses.   *Bull.   WHO* **29,**   7–41, 1963.

Hackett, C.   An International Nomenclature of Yaws Lesions.   *WHO* Monogr. 36, 103 pp., 1957.

Horsfall, F., and Tamm, I.   *Viral and Rickettsial Infections of Man.*   Philadelphia, Lippincott, 1965.

VI

22 Tropical Ophthalmology

Blindness, a personal tragedy in any country, is both an individual and a family disaster in the tropics. When vision is lost, the ability to hunt, farm or labour is lost also; it becomes impossible to provide for one's self or dependants or to avoid the assaults of wild animals and the constant threat of accidents. Blindness is prevalent throughout the tropics; the fact that most of it is caused either by ignorance or by preventable and treatable infections compounds the tragedy. In addition to the lesions which are known to cause blindness in temperate climates also, there are a number of aetiological factors peculiar to the tropics. Smallpox, onchocerciasis, loiasis, leprosy, South American leishmaniasis, rickettsioses, malaria and dengue are discussed elsewhere in this book. By far the most significant ophthalmologic malady in the tropics is trachoma. Although this virus infection might have been included in Part IV of this text, it is more logically discussed here so that various eye lesions can be considered together as alternatives in differential diagnosis.

TRACHOMA

Trachoma is a chronic viral disease affecting the conjunctiva and the cornea. Almost one sixth of the world's population, 500 million persons, are victims of trachoma. However, the severity of the disease varies greatly and is as much related to environmental conditions as to susceptibility of the host and differences in strains of the virus. For example, trachoma is a far more virulent disease in the hot, dry, crowded area of the Middle East than it is in the moist farmlands of interior Taiwan.

The aetiological virus is a member of the psittacosis–lymphogranuloma group. Whereas it can now be both isolated and cultured the virus had been recognized for many years as the intracytoplasmic

170

inclusions—Halberstaedter–Prowazek (H–P) bodies—seen in scrapings from the upper tarsal conjunctiva of trachoma patients.

Clinical and pathological features. After an incubation period of from 2 to 12 days the virus multiplies on the upper tarsal surface and causes progressive epithelial proliferation, follicle formation, papillary hypertrophy and, eventually, pannus formation and cicatrization. As scarring progresses, trichiasis (inversion of a lash) or entropion (lid inversion) occurs, with resultant corneal ulceration or total obliteration by the pannus. As scarring continues and involves the limbal follicles, transparent epithelium fills the retracted defects, causing pathogno-monic Herbert's peripheral pits. Secondary bacterial infection is common; in fact, most uncomplicated trachoma infections are self-limiting; it is the bacterial contaminants that often cause severe damage.

The early clinical patterns range from the asymptomatic to one with ptosis and acute conjunctivitis. Examination of the everted upper eyelid reveals the extent of damage (MacCallum's classification) with minimal follicles found in stage I, hypertrophic follicles and papillae in stage II, and pannus and scar tissue in advanced (stage III) cases. Stage IV refers to healed trachoma with the conjunctiva completely cicatrized and without follicles or papillae (Figs. 76 and 77).

Diagnosis may be confirmed by visualization of H–P bodies, by culture of the virus on chick embryo sacs or by serological and immuno-fluorescent techniques. In the field, clinical diagnosis is acceptable; in an American or a European city, laboratory confirmation would be essential.

Treatment. The virus is sensitive to sulpha and some antibiotic drugs. Recommended regimen for the treatment of an acute case is as follows:

(1) A long-acting sulpha drug such as sulphamethoxypyridazine in an adult oral dosage of 3 g daily for 3 weeks.

(2) Local antibiotic therapy with tetracycline ophthalmic ointment.

(3) Specific treatment of secondary bacterial contaminants. Surgical correction of advanced lid inversion is often necessary.

Trachoma vaccine trials are still in the experimental stage.

SPARGANOSIS

Indigenous medical practice in the tropics is based more on super-stition than on fact, and the patient who recovers frequently does so in spite of therapy. The topical use of poultices is a common prescription to 'draw out the disease'. One such regimen, the application of fresh

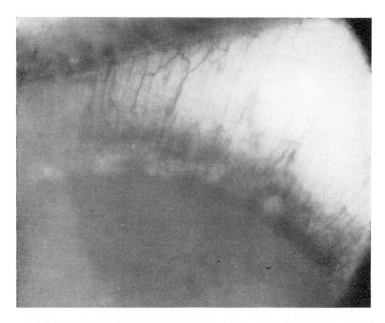

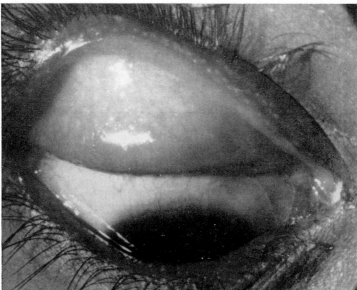

Fig. 76. Trachoma. *Top*, early limbal follicles and typical vascular pattern in stage I. *Bottom*, prominent follicular hypertrophy on the upper tarsus and early corneal pannus in stage II.

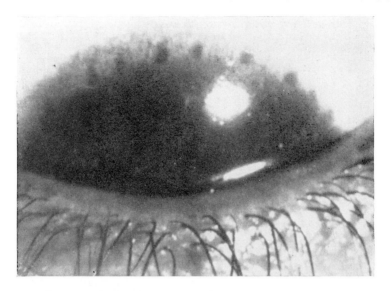

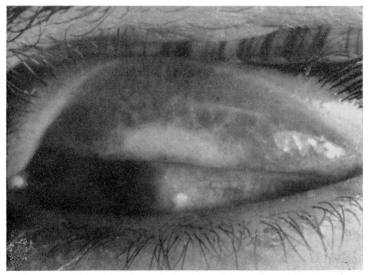

Fig. 77. Trachoma *cont.* *Top*, well-developed Herbert's peripheral pits and pannus. *Bottom*, fine horizontal scars, Arlt's lines in end-stage, cicatrized trachoma.

frog meat to sore eyes, is a frequent cause of ocular damage in the Far East. Though the custom rarely cures anyone, it does permit the plerocercoid form of a parasite of the frog, *Diphyllobothrium mansoni* or sparganum, to migrate into the warmer human tissue and cause irritation, corneal ulceration, nodule formation and secondary infection. Ocular sparganosis can result in unilateral blindness. Diagnosis of the eye lesion is possible only by incising the tumours and finding the parasite. Therapy is unsatisfactory; the parasite must first be killed with alcohol or novarsobenzol and then either removed surgically or allowed to reabsorb gradually. Generalized sparganosis may follow the drinking of water contaminated with cyclops harbouring another intermediate form of the parasite.

MALNUTRITION AND EYE DISEASE

It is as difficult to correlate defective vision with malnutrition as it is to determine the general effect of diet on disease. However, several specific nutritional deficiencies are known to cause eye damage. The most serious of these is hypovitaminosis A. Vitamin A is required for the deposition of rhodopsin in the rods of the retina and for the preservation of healthy epithelial cells. An estimated 20,000 children are blinded annually with these lesions. Inadequate—and even zero—serum levels of vitamin A are common in children throughout the tropics, since foods containing either preformed vitamin A or carotene precursors are rare dietary items.

In infants with levels of vitamin A that are barely sufficient to prevent ophthalmopathological complications, illnesses such as acute diarrhoea, in which there is rapid intestinal movement and decreased fat absorption, leave the child dependent on hepatic vitamin A stores. As protein deficiency develops, even these stores—if there were any—cannot be mobilized.

Reversible retinal lesions evidenced by night blindness and detected by rod scotometry are the earliest signs of hypovitaminosis A. Drying of the conjunctival surface with local keratin deposits on the surface (Bitot's spots) follows. The cornea becomes xerotic, necrotic and ulcerated. Permanent loss of vision may be related to panophthalmitis, iris incarceration or lens extrusion.

If treatment with parenteral and oral vitamin A (total dose of 100,000 IU) is begun before the keratomalacia stage, complete and rapid recovery occurs. However, surgical correction or orbital extraction is often necessary once colliquative necrosis has begun. Prevention is readily accomplished by enhancing diets with rich sources of vitamin A, such as cod liver oil or red palm oil, or by providing concentrated vitamin tablets or drops through maternal and child welfare clinics in endemic areas.

Vitamin B deficiencies were frequently a cause of visual disturbances among malnourished prisoners of war in World War II. Thiamine and riboflavin deficiencies were primarily responsible for the early photo-phobia and the late irreversible optic atrophy that characterized Far Eastern 'nutritional amblyopia'.

HAEMOGLOBINOPATHIES

Thromboses are common complications of various haemoglobin-opathies; their occurrence in sickle-cell disease is well known to most clinicians. Retinal thromboses are noted particularly in patients who have a combination of Haemoglobin S and Haemoglobin C; the latter is a variant of high incidence in north Ghana. Haemoglobin C cells sickle at a lower oxygen tension than do S-S cells. The anaemia is not as severe in S-C disease as in S-S; ironically, it is this absence of anaemia that may be the explanation for the high proportion of blinding retinal thromboses. A densely packed, relatively viscid blood supply will stagnate on a few sickled cells in the narrow lumen of an arteriole more easily than will a thin, anaemic stream. Patients often experience multiple episodes of transient amblyopia or amaurosis. Both retinal haemorrhages and pallor can be seen by ophthalmoscopy. Treatment is limited to anticoagulation. Patients with S-C disease should be advised to avoid low oxygen tensions such as occur in high-altitude, unpressurized flying.

IATROGENIC FACTORS

The eye lesions related to tropical diseases that will be seen most commonly by the temperate-climate clinician will be those caused by him or his colleagues. Iatrogenic eye damage can result from a wide variety of drugs in common use for the treatment or the prevention of tropical diseases. The more important compounds incriminated are the synthetic antimalarials, quinine and the arsenicals.

VI

Synthetic antimalarials. All of the synthetic antimalarials are oculotoxic if they are administered in high doses for long periods. This is rarely, if ever, a problem in the routine treatment or prevention of malaria; most reports of eye damage due to synthetic antimalarials follow intensive administration in the treatment of collagen diseases. For example, in the management of systemic lupus erythematosus, 750 mg of chloroquine (one half the *total* dose for the radical cure of malaria) may be administered daily for years. Under these conditions accommodation defects, diplopia, corneal deposits, subcapsular opacities, keratopathy and severe retinopathy, including arteriolar narrowing, and aberrant pigmentation, especially in the macular area, are common. The corneal lesions are reversible on discontinuation of the drug; the retinal lesions are usually permanent. Neither should result from properly managed prophylaxis or treatment of malaria.

Quinine is still used widely for the treatment and the prevention of malaria. As chloroquine-resistance became a major problem in Southeast Asia and South America, quinine and the syndrome cinchonism, the toxic reaction to the drug, became, once again, a clinical challenge. Cinchonism usually occurs only after excessively long regimens or excessively high doses of quinine have been administered, but it may be an idiosyncratic reaction to a single tablet. Amblyopia and amaurosis usually are transient, disappearing within the 72 hours required for total drug excretion. However, permanent blindness or tubular vision occurs occasionally. Ophthalmoscopy may reveal retinal artery spasm, ischaemia and oedema with pallor of the discs and optic atrophy. Emergency treatment of the ocular aspects of acute cinchonism includes intravenous papaverine or sodium nitrate for arterial dilatation.

Arsenical drugs are used widely in the treatment of trypanosomiasis and, occasionally, in the management of patients with amoebiasis and filariasis. Oculotoxic reactions to both trivalent and pentavalent compounds are common; for example, 10 per cent of patients who receive a full course of tryparsamide note visual changes. Usually, these are limited to transient eye pain, photophobia, lacrimorrhoea and defects in focusing and light adaptation. Concentric contraction of the visual field with a central scotoma is a characteristic toxic reaction of a more serious nature. The latter vanishes within a few days if the drug is withdrawn promptly, but peripheral field defects are often permanent. If the drug is continued in spite of early toxic signs, the victim frequently becomes totally and permanently blind. In western medical centres, where the use of arsenicals for tropical diseases is rare, where facilities for adequate examinations are or can be available, and where the pressures of mass treatment as a public health measure do not exist, visual acuity and field studies should be done before, during and after a regimen of tryparsamide. British antilewisite (BAL) should always be available. As noted in the chapter on African Trypanosomiasis, BAL is now combined with the arsenicals as Mel B; though toxicity is thereby reduced, the danger of ocular damage remains.

MECHANICAL FACTORS

The direct effects of wind and dirt in arid areas are largely responsible for the prevalence of pterygium in the tropics. As this corneal growth occludes the pupil, visual loss follows; surgical removal of the pterygium is the only effective therapy.

Glare conjunctivitis is another danger in the bright desert areas of the tropics. The conjunctiva is desquamated by ultraviolet rays, producing an excruciating blindness. Treatment includes topical use of atropine and cocaine and rest in a dark room; antibiotics are often indicated to control secondary infection. Patients who plan to visit the tropics should be advised to bring polaroid or reflecting sunglasses.

The final, and perhaps the most important, cause of eye damage in the tropics defies exact classification. The roles of ignorance, filth and neglect in the aetiology of tropical blindness are complex; they may be primary causes, and they are, unfortunately, almost always complicating factors. Their elimination will depend—as do almost all advances in tropical medicine—on general improvements in education, social and personal hygiene and water distribution, as well as on an expansion of medical and public health facilities and knowledge.

BIBLIOGRAPHY

T'ang, F., Chang, H., Huang, Y., and Wang, K.   Studies on the Etiology of Trachoma. *Chinese med. J.* **75,** 429, 1957.
Tarizzo, M., and Nataf, R.   The Treatment of Trachoma.   *Rev. int. Trachome* **46,** 7, 1970.
Roger, F., and Sinclair, H.   *Metabolic and Nutritional Eye Diseases.*   Springfield, Ill., Charles C. Thomas, 419 pp., 1969.
Henkind, P., and Rothfield, N.   Ocular Abnormalities in Patients Treated with Synthetic Antimalarial Drugs.   *New Engl. J. Med.* **269,** 433, 1963.
Somerset, E. J.   *Ophthalmology in the Tropics.*   London, Baillière, Tindall and Cox, 1962.

VII

23 Miscellaneous Tropical Diseases

The use of the term Exotic Diseases as a synonym for Tropical Medicine is particularly appropriate in regard to those epidemic illnesses of unknown aetiology and bizarre symptomatology that are confined to local areas within the tropics. They will rarely, if ever, present a diagnostic or therapeutic challenge to the physician in a temperate climate, but a knowledge of these diseases is often essential for the full understanding of related maladies.

EFFECTS OF HEAT

Throughout the tropics indigenous patterns of diet, activity, clothing and housing assist man's physiological adaptation to high levels of heat and humidity. Because of ignorance or the pressures of organized trips, the modern tourist has altered the old saying that only 'mad dogs and Englishmen' go out in the noonday sun.

The body's reaction to thermal stress is influenced by the duration of exposure, the humidity, the air velocity, the amount and the type of radiant heat, exercise and clothing as well as by the dry bulb temperature. Man responds to an effective temperature rise by vasodilatation, increased sweating and conservation of salt and water by an increased output of antidiuretic hormone and aldosterone. Water loss from sweating alone may exceed 10 litres per day. In the desert a person may lose 7 per cent of his body weight and 30 g of sodium chloride in a day. Acclimatization to the high effective temperatures of the tropics is partial and gradual. Studies on subjects in the deserts of Arabia and in the stifling mines of South Africa have demonstrated the need for exposure of at least several weeks' duration before the ability to tolerate high effective temperatures is improved. The average tourist or victim of a local hot spell will have had no chance for physiological adaptation.

In fact, probably the most common ailment of Caucasians first visiting the tropics is severe sunburn secondary to injudicious exposure to the bright sun with inadequate protective clothing and insufficient time to develop a tan.

Reactions to thermal stress may be either minor or major. The former include prickly heat, or thermogenic anhidrosis, and heat cramps. The flow of sweat in the patient with prickly heat is blocked and the swollen glands produce a papular eruption, mammillaria, on the covered parts of the body. The skin is warm and dry, salt depletion is rare, and the major danger is that the condition predisposes to collapse with hyperpyrexia if exposure to heat is continued.

Heat hyperpyrexia (or heatstroke) is the most serious reaction to high effective temperatures. Studies on the aetiology and the pathology of this syndrome are complex; it is sufficient for our purposes to understand that those who are most commonly afflicted are the unacclimatized who have exhausted their sweating mechanism. Then, as the demands for perspiration are not met, the skin becomes warm and dry, the heat-regulating centres of the hypothalamus are damaged and a vicious cycle of hyperpyrexia to 110°F with decreased sweating ensues. The patient may pass through an agitated, violent stage, followed by lassitude, confusion and coma. If sweating has not resumed within 12 hours the outcome is invariably fatal. Prognosis is directly correlated with age, degree of hyperpyrexia, duration of symptoms, the presence or the absence of coma, and the rapidity with which treatment is begun. Those who survive usually have had the benefits of prompt and effective therapy; this primarily involves cooling, which may be accomplished by submersion in cool water, water-sponging and massaging under constant fanning, or the use of air-conditioning.

Intravenous chlorpromazine is a valuable addition to the mechanical measures because of its thermolytic and sedative properties. Serum electrolytes and urinary chlorides are normal in patients with heatstroke, and fluid replacement should be limited to a slow intravenous drip of 5 per cent dextrose and saline. The most crucial differential diagnosis in heat hyperpyrexia is cerebral malaria. If there is any question of falciparum infection in a hyperpyrexic individual, intramuscular chloroquine should be added to the regimen. Patients who plan strenuous activities in the tropics should be advised of the need for loose clothing and adequate available fluids and, especially, of the danger incurred if they exhaust their sweating mechanisms by prolonged exposure to heat before they start work.

The other major reaction to a torrid effective temperature is heat exhaustion. This syndrome is due to an excessive loss of sodium chloride through copious sweating and inadequate electrolyte replacement. As extracellular dehydration becomes marked or is corrected only by replacement with water, cardiovascular collapse ensues. The skin is cool and clammy; the blood pressure is reduced; the body temperature is normal or only slightly elevated and the sensorium is clear. Serum chlorides are diminished, urinary chlorides are absent, blood urea is elevated, and there may be oliguria with marked albuminuria. Treatment is based on rapid replacement of fluids and electrolytes. The first 500 ml of 5 per cent dextrose and saline should be administered in 10 minutes, and the second in 20 minutes. Intravenous fluids should be continued until blood pressure is maintained and the urinary flow exceeds 2 litres. Obviously, it is essential to monitor fluid replacement by careful clinical examinations in order to avoid overtransfusion. There is no reason to cool patients with heat exhaustion; in fact, moderate warming with blankets is both desirable and comforting to the patient. Persons who expect to be exposed to hot, humid climates should be advised to wear loose clothing, to imbibe water freely, especially while performing muscular work, and to be sure to maintain an adequate salt intake. This usually can be accomplished by increasing dietary salt from 10 to 30 g per day; inclusion of extra salt in fruit drinks is one palatable means. Many types of salt tablets are commercially available for those whose need to replace salt losses is particularly heavy and constant.

KURU

In 1957 a new neurological disorder was described among the aboriginal Fore tribe of remote western New Guinea. Since that time the cases of more than 5,000 victims of kuru have been intensively investigated, and, though the clinical, the pathological and the epidemiological patterns of the disease are now well described, the aetiology remains uncertain and the mortality exceeds 90 per cent. A slow-acting, latent virus has been incriminated. The disease, which afflicts male or female children and adult women, has an insidious onset marked by clumsiness. The patient develops ataxia, athetosis, dysarthria, dysphagia, marked emotional lability and, in the final, bed-ridden stage, nutritional deficiencies, decubiti and bronchopneumonia. Death within a year is the rule.

The disease is as perplexing to the pathologist as it is to the clinician.

Diffuse nonspecific neuronal degeneration is found throughout the mid-brain. The results of cerebrospinal fluid examination, haemogram, biochemical analyses for heavy metals and investigations for bacterial, rickettsial and protozoal agents have been normal. The hypotheses of a genetic aetiology and of an autoimmune mechanism are being investigated. The relationship of kuru to scrapie in sheep and to disseminated or multiple sclerosis in man has stimulated reinvestigation of the pathogenesis of these diseases. There is no known treatment for kuru.

AINHUM

Ainhum is a rare disease of Africans and their descendants in the Americas and Asia, in which progressive fissure formation and fibrosis occur at a terminal phalangeal joint. The little toe is the usual site, but ainhum of the fingers also has been reported. The disease is first noted as a crease in the digitoplantar fold, and a sulcus with cicatrized borders gradually develops. As the fissure deepens, a constricting fibrous band isolates the terminal phalanx from the digit and dry gangrene with spontaneous amputation occurs (dactylolysis spontanea). The aetiology of this bizarre affliction is unknown; the most common theories have been those related to trauma, keloid formation, yaws, leprosy, syphilis and collagen diseases. An operation, Z-plasty, has been successful in the treatment of early lesions, but amputation is necessary in advanced cases.

TROPICAL SPRUE

Physicians who treat Americans or Europeans are more likely to encounter tropical sprue than are local doctors in the tropics who work with indigenous populations. Tropical sprue is a disease of uncertain aetiology which afflicts recent visitors to coastal areas of India, the Far East and the Caribbean. It is one of the malabsorption syndromes and presents clinically with the typical features of steatorrhoea, diarrhoea, abdominal distention, flatus, weight loss, weakness, glossitis, hypotension and, occasionally, megaloblastic anaemia. The skin is pale and dry; a dusky hue is often noticeable on the cheeks and the forehead of light-skinned patients. The faeces of a patient with tropical sprue are bulky, greasy and pale.

Frequently, the first bowel movement of the day will awaken the patient at about 4 or 5 a.m.; after this, there may be four or five explosive movements before noontime, with complete cessation as the day progresses. The disease is remitting, but, if it is untreated over long periods, the patient almost invariably becomes debilitated.

A wide range of laboratory tests are available to assess the aetiology and the extent of pathology in malabsorption syndromes. In tropical sprue, as in the nontropical variety, jejunal biopsy will reveal flattened villi. Barium will clump in the nonmotile, excess mucosa of the bowel. The levels of fat-soluble vitamins are low, and the fat content of the stool is increased. Intestinal absorption is deranged as measured by tolerance tests of glucose, xylose or vitamin A.

Treatment during the acute phase should be begun with bed rest in a hospital. The change in environment may itself initiate improvement; return to a temperate climate from the endemic zone is almost always associated with a cure. A low-carbohydrate, low-fat, high-protein diet with supplementary calcium and B-complex vitamins is indicated. Spicy foods and alcohol are strictly interdicted. Megaloblastic anaemia, when it is found, responds to administration of folic acid. Broad-spectrum antibiotics appear to be effective in certain patients with tropical sprue, but the mechanism of action is not understood.

BIBLIOGRAPHY

Browne, S. G. Ainhum: A Clinical and Etiological Study of 63 Cases. *Ann. trop. Med. Parasit.* **55,** 314, 1961.
Gajdusek, D. Kuru. *Trans. R. Soc. trop. Med. Hyg.* **57,** 151, 1963.
Leithead, C., and Lind, A. *Heat Stress and Heat Disorders*. London, Cassell, 1963.
Garbach, S. (ed.). A Symposium on Tropical Sprue. *Am. J. clin. Nutr.* **23,** 1545–81, 1970.

VIII

---

24 Advising the Tropical Traveller

The number of tourists and businessmen who visit the tropics is many times greater today than it was even a decade ago. Most travellers must see a physician occasionally to comply with immunization requirements, but those who are going to the torrid zone have greater reason to seek medical advice and are more likely to do so. Therefore, the practitioner must be acquainted with the endemic zones of major quarantinable diseases. He must be aware of the potential protection that is available to his patient through vaccinations, prophylactic medications and advice on sanitation and insect control, as well as through preliminary medical instruction in regard to the pitfalls of diet that so commonly spoil sojourns. The physician must be able to provide a medical kit of essential items for those who intend to venture far from urban centres (Table 13). By giving the patient a copy of pertinent data from his medical record, together with advice on measures to be taken should illness occur in a foreign town, the practitioner will do much to allay the anxieties of the tropical traveller. The doctor must be prepared to re-examine the patient on his return and to evaluate any findings in light of the areas which were visited. I have reviewed this topic, in much greater detail than is possible here, in the book noted in the Bibliography.

PRIOR TO DEPARTURE

The first need, and often a recurrent one, of many prospective tropical travellers is reassurance. The theatrical concept of the tropics as a vast, primitive area where all wilt in the noonday sun and life is preserved by oral infusions of gin and tonic should be dispelled. Adequate food and lodging, good hospitals and competent clinicians with a knowledge of English are available in every major tropical town. Although the heat

Table 13. The medical kit

ALL TRAVELLERS
1 Personal physician's report and telephone number
2 Red Cross first aid booklet
3 Assorted bandages, cotton, scissors, tweezers, thermometer, flat toilet paper, sunburn lotion
4 Aspirin
5 Antihistamines: Chlortrimeton; Benadryl
6 Pills for motion sickness
7 Paregoric
8 Antibiotics (tetracycline)
9 Sleeping pills

TROPICAL TRAVELLERS
10 Analgesics: codeine; demerol
11 Disposable needles and syringes
12 Salt tablets
13 Insect repellents
14 Mosquito net
15 Antimalarials (chloroquine)
16 Water-purification tablets
17 Soap

can be excessive and the high humidity or the rains may be oppressive at times, the careful tourist can avoid these extremes by planning to make his trip during the clear seasons. Air-conditioning is available in most of the hotels that the average tourist is likely to frequent. Persons who plan to spend long periods in the tropics must adapt mentally, as they will physiologically, to torrid zones. It should be noted that mentally unstable persons may break under the strain of cultural differences and monotonous heat or rain. Therefore, those who require constant medical supervision for either a mental or a physical condition should be advised not to go to the tropics unless preliminary arrangements for suitable therapy there have been completed.

The same diseases that afflict man in temperate climates can complicate a tropical tour. The practitioner can serve both his patient and his tropical medical colleague by furnishing an account (to be carried in the same special wallet with passport, travellers' cheques and vaccination certificate) of the status of the traveller's health on departure. Those with chronic illnesses such as diabetes, epilepsy and coronary artery disease should be made aware of the danger signals of relapse and urged to seek local medical supervision. Patients who require regular medication should be given a supply of drugs adequate for the whole trip before departure; a list of all medicines, with generic and trade names as well as dosages, should be included in the physician's summary. It may be advisable to include pertinent laboratory data, especially a recent electrocardiogram for patients with ischaemic heart disease. Finally, the physician's office telephone number should be provided in case the patient or the tropical doctor should seek emergency advice and information.

The prospective traveller should be reassured when he learns that, although the exotic diseases endemic in the tropics are serious illnesses which can be fatal, most of them are preventable by the use of immunizations, prophylactic medications and common sense. For example, insect-borne diseases may be effectively avoided by the wearing of sensible clothing, such as trousers and long-sleeved shirts, and by the use of mosquito netting at night and insecticides in houses or insect repellents in the open. Additional protection in malarious areas is advisable. As in the treatment of malaria, so also in prophylaxis, chloroquine is the preferred drug; 300 mg of the base once weekly is the prophylactic adult dose. The drug should be taken on entering a malarious area and continued for at least 4 weeks after leaving the endemic region. Since protective blood levels are obtained within hours of taking chloroquine, it is no longer necessary to begin prophylaxis 10 days before arrival, as it was when mepacrine was widely used. After departure the traveller should also take primaquine in a daily dosage of 15 mg for 2 weeks.

Pentamidine prophylaxis against African trypanosomiasis is not recommended. Even though it has been stated that a single injection of 200 mg offers considerable protection for 3 to 4 months, the facts are that risk of infection for the average visitor are minimal; that incomplete protection is extremely dangerous, since it may mask the early, treatable lesions; and that low blood levels of pentamidine can promote the emergence of drug-resistant trypanosomes.

IMMUNIZATIONS

Protection against a wide range of diseases can be obtained by inoculation procedures, and, in this regard, the tropical traveller in particular deserves careful attention (Table 14). Smallpox vaccination within 3 years is still demanded by many countries. Although the United States has eliminated smallpox requirements for visitors from most parts of the world, other nations are not bound by this move. One of the

Table 14. Primary inoculations for tropical travellers

Disease	Dosage*	Efficacy	Contraindications	Side effects	Protective within (days)	Protective for (years)
Smallpox	Multiple pressure	4+	<6 months' age Pregnancy Skin disease	Encephalitis Vaccinia generalized gangrenosa	Primary: 8 Revaccin: immed.	3
Yellow Fever	0·5 ml, s.c.	4+	<6 months' age Pregnancy	17–D: none Dakar: encephalitis, fever	10	10
Cholera	0·5 ml, s.c. then 1·0 ml, s.c.	1–2+	0	Local erythema and oedema	6	1/2
Typhoid	0·5 ml × 2, s.c. or 0·1 ml × 2, i.d.	3+	0	Local erythema and oedema, 12 fever		1
Tetanus–Diphtheria	0·5 ml, s.c.	4+	0	Mild erythema and oedema		5
Typhus (strain E)	1·0 ml × 2, s.c.	3+	Marked egg sensitivity	Local erythema and oedema	14	1
Poliomyelitis	Sabin	4+	0	0	14	(?)5+
Hepatitis	4 cc gamma globulin	3+	0	0	Immed.	1/2
Plague	1·0 ml × 3, s.c.	1–2+	0	Local erythema and oedema Fever, vomiting, chills, rigor	6	1/2

* See text for booster doses

most important reasons a traveller should have his inoculation booklet up to date and properly certified is to avoid unnecessary hardship at a foreign port. It often seems that there is an inverse ratio between the size of the airport or country and the amount of attention devoted to apparently insignificant minutiae such as the certification stamp on immunization booklets. The method, the classification, the contra-indications and the complications of smallpox vaccination have been reviewed earlier. It should be stressed that, when a contraindication exists, medical reasons should be stated clearly on professional station-ery. Foreign governments *may* accept exemptions, but they can impose quarantine restrictions if indications are adequate.

Poliomyelitis, tetanus, typhoid and diphtheria are prevalent through-out the tropics and all travellers should be protected against them; none of these vaccinations is required by law. Since the typhoid in-jections must be separated by 10 days and since febrile reactions to the vaccine occur, it is important to begin this series well in advance of the planned date of departure. The injections should be given in the late afternoon, if possible, so that the reaction will occur mainly during sleep. A moderate analgesic such as aspirin or codeine (gr $\frac{1}{4}$) will alleviate some of the untoward reactions. The phenolized typhoid vaccine has proved 80 per cent protective in a wide-scale WHO field trial, whereas the alcohol-killed vaccine has been shown to be in-effective. The para A and para B components of the old TAB vaccine have been eliminated since they were not only ineffective but respon-sible for much of the untoward reactions. Inoculations may be either subcutaneous or intradermal.

Almost all children and the majority of adults (either in the Armed Forces or at the time of a previous accident) have received tetanus inoculations. If less than 10 years have passed since inoculation, a 'booster' dose of 0·5 ml of the toxoid will elicit a protective response. The Sabin polio vaccine elicits a greater antibody response and is my choice for the most effective polio protection in the tropics. Immuniza-tion against diphtheria and pertussis is safe and effective in children and should certainly be done before visiting the tropics. Diphtheria inoculation of adults with the purified preparations now available is no longer associated with the severe local and systemic reactions that previously contraindicated its use. It is not necessary now to perform Schick and Moloney tests to indicate the need for and the safety of inoculation.

Visitors to the endemic zones in Africa and the Americas should receive yellow fever vaccinations. Most of the nations in the endemic belt demand a certificate of vaccination dated at least 10 days before arrival, and many countries require vaccination of all persons over the age of 6 months on re-entry from infected areas. Reactions are rare and minimal. There is no validity to the old requirement of imposing a 14-day delay between smallpox and yellow fever inoculations.

Although the immunity stimulated by cholera vaccination is often unsatisfactory, it is an advisable protection for any visitor to endemic zones. Two injections are needed, mild systemic reactions are common, and a 'booster' is necessary every 6 months. A certificate of vaccination is required for entry into most Asiatic and African countries, and wherever there has recently been an outbreak. Plague vaccination is not required by law by any country, and, since severe reactions are common and the protection short-lived, only when exposure is likely should immunization be advised. Typhus vaccination also is not required by any country today. Only those persons who may expect to enter lousy and poor areas of infected zones require vaccination. Separate, killed vaccines against louse-borne typhus and flea-borne typhus are available but neither protect against scrub or mite-borne typhus. The live vaccine of strain E of *Rickettsia prowazeki* is the most effective typhus vaccine available and does provide cross-protection for murine typhus.

After all the attention to dramatic tropical infections, it must be remembered that one of the most frequent acquisitions of the casual traveller is hepatitis. This is the most common physical cause for medical evacuation of missionaries, volunteer workers and diplomats from the tropics. Since the disability from hepatitis is measured in months rather than days or weeks, every possible protection should be sought. Avoidance of faecal contamination directly or in water and food is most important. Passive immunization with gamma globulin is recommended. An adult dosage of 4 cc intramuscularly will reduce the clinical incidence of infectious hepatitis by some 80 per cent. The protection is short-lived, lasting only 4 to 6 months.

The physician has a great array of immunization procedures available for the protection of his travelling patient; some are recommended for all patients, while others should be selected only for those visiting endemic areas. To repeat routinely a full course of typhoid or tetanus injections for those with previous inoculations or to inflict yellow fever, typhus and plague vaccines on the tourist who intends to visit Japan causes needless suffering. Table 14 summarizes the dosages and the protection elicited by the various immunizations.

THE TRIP

The first experience of many travellers on a long-awaited trip is, unfortunately, nausea. Motion sickness, together with anxiety attendant on flying or sailing and departure, can be allayed by a wide variety of compounds. Although comparative drug studies are wanting, effective agents include anti-emetics, such as meclazine hydrochloride and its derivatives, and primary sedatives such as the barbiturates. Both are mildly soporific. This may be of advantage to the weary air passenger, but it may be dangerous if attentive observation, such as is required in business conferences or driving, is required within 12 hours. Sea journeys on most large liners have been made more comfortable by hydrofoil stabilizers. The sanitary facilities of all major international vessels are controlled by international agreements, and travellers should be equally reassured in regard to the safety of food and water on board.

THE TROPICS

The same cannot be said for much of the food and the water in the tropics. Even in the major cities and hotels caution must be exercised, since native cooks and food-handlers are frequently carriers of disease, adherence to common sanitary practices is sporadic, if not nonexistent, and adequate refrigeration and food preservation are the exceptions rather than the rule. Pastries, custards, cold meat and buffet platters and leafy salads must be strictly avoided. Fresh fruits with unbroken skin may be eaten after peeling, and fully cooked or canned foods are safe. Soaking of vegetables in potassium permanganate or chlorine solutions is not protective.

Milk should always be boiled, since bovine tuberculosis and brucellosis are common veterinary diseases. Water should be purified before drinking, either by boiling or by chemical methods. A chlorinated halazone tablet will sterilize a quart of water in 30 minutes. Unbottled soft drinks may not be pure, but most alcoholic beverages can be consumed (in moderation) safely. By following these simple precautions the gourmet can savour the majority of tropical delicacies and yet avoid the prostrating dysentery and other diseases that have been noted. There is no effective drug prophylaxis against amoebic infection, and observation of the above recommendations is the best protection. A transient diarrhoea—'tourista', or 'gippy'—complicates many tropical trips. The cause of this syndrome remains obscure and the use of antibiotic prophylactics does not reduce the incidence.

Patients who plan to visit schistosomal zones should be warned against bathing in freshwater canals, rivers and lakes. Canals throughout the tropics harbour leptospira. Casual contact with animals (including household pets) should be avoided. Not only is rabies rife in the tropics but many animals serve as intermediate vectors of parasitic infections. I do not suggest routine rabies inoculations for travellers.

If a patient should become ill and require medical attention, the major hotels, the offices of the major transportation lines and the embassies or consulates of the United States, United Kingdom, France, Germany, for instance, can provide a list of physicians. Those whose graduate qualification or training has been obtained in a major western centre are most likely to have the adequate command of both English and medicine that is necessary to provide the type of care required.

ON RETURN

At the conclusion of the tropical tour, the patient should return to his physician for re-examination. This should include a sigmoidoscopy, especially if the traveller experienced diarrhoea during his time overseas. An eosinophil count, thick and thin blood smears and a stool examination for ova and parasites are useful survey techniques if complete reassurance is desired. In view of the long incubation period of many helminthic infections, a second stool examination 3 months after return may be made. The development of parasitic serology is a major advance for the rapid screening of large numbers of travellers to the tropics exposed to a wide range of 'exotic' infections that, once again, must be part of the good clinician's differential diagnosis throughout the temperate climates.

BIBLIOGRAPHY

Cahill, K. *Medical Advice for the Traveler.* New York, Holt, Rinehart and Winston, 79 pp., 1970; paperback, *Popular Library*, 1972.
Ross Institute of Tropical Hygiene. *Preservation of Personal Health in Warm Climates.* London, 7th edn, 102 pp., 1971, reprinted 1973.
American Society of Tropical Medicine and Hygiene. *Health Hints for the Tropics*, 6th edn, 31 pp., 1967.
Rule, C. *A Traveler's Guide to Good Health.* New York, Doubleday and Co., 166 pp., 1960.

INDEX

Index

A

Aedes aegypti, vector in arbor virus
  infections 153, 154, 158–9
  filariasis 69, 77
  yellow fever 152–5, 157
A. africanus, simpsoni, vectors in yellow
  fever 153, 154
African trypanosomiasis (sleeping
    sickness) 27–35
  clinical features 31–2
  diagnosis 32–4
  distribution 27–8
  Glossina species, vectors 29
  Kerandel's sign 32
  pathological features 29–30
  protozoal forms 28–9, 32
  treatment 34–5
  tsetse fly *see Glosinia* above
  Winterbottom's sign 32
ainhum 181
Alcopar *see* bephenium
    hydroxynaphthoate
alveolar hydatid disease *see*
    echinococcosis
Ambilhar *see* niridazole
American trypanosomiasis (Chigas
    disease) 35–41
  'assassin' or 'kissing' bug *see*
    Triatoma
  cardiac signs 36–8
  clinical features 38–9
  distribution and incidence 35
  life cycle of *Trypanosoma cruzi* 35–6
  Machado–Guerreiro test 40
  megacolon 39
  pathological features 35–7
  Romaña's sign 37, 38
  treatment 40–1
  Triatoma (reduviid) bugs 35, 36, 38
amoebiasis 14–27
  clinical features 19–20

complications
  amoeboma 20, 23
  appendicitis 20
  liver abscess 19, 20, 23, 26
  lung abscess 20
  perforation 19–20
diagnosis 20–4
Entamoeba histolytica 14–15, 20–3,
    25–6
giardiasis 27
pathological features 15, 19
prevention 26, 189
treatment 27
anaemia in
  African trypanosomiasis 30
  bartonellosis 145
  Diphyllobothrium latum infection 126
  hookworm 64–5, 66, 68
  malaria 7, 8
  schistosomiasis 108
  tropical sprue 181–2
  visceral leishmaniasis 43
  yellow fever 156
Ancylostoma braziliensis and *A. caninum*
    in larva migrans 93
A. duodenale see hookworm
Anopheles, vector in filariasis, 68, 77
  malaria 1, 7
antimony compounds, use in
    leishmaniasis 45, 47
  schistosomiasis 102, 107, 109
Antrypol *see* suramin
arbor virus infections 152–9
Argentinian haemorrhagic fever 154
Arlt's lines *see* trachoma
arsenicals
  ocular toxicity 34, 176–7
  use in
    amoebiasis 26
    trypanosomiasis 34, 176–7
Arsobal *see* Mel B

arthropod-borne viruses *see* arbor virus infections
ascariasis 87–90
'assassin' bug *see* American trypanosomiasis
Astiban (TWSB), use in schistosomiasis 102
Atabrine *see* quinacrine hydrochloride

B

bacterial diseases 127–45
Balantium coli 17
bartonellosis 142–3, 145
Bayer 7602, use in American trypanosomiasis 40–1
BCG, use of, in
  leprosy 135
  toxoplasmosis 62
beef tapeworm *see* Taeniasis saginata
bejel *see* yaws
bephenium hydroxynaphthoate, use in hookworm 67
bilharziasis *see* schistosomiasis
Bithionol, use in paragonimiasis 121
Bitot's spots in hypovitaminosis A 174
'black fever' *see* visceral leishmaniasis
blackwater fever in malaria 8, 11, 13
brucellosis, danger of 189
Brugia malayi see filariasis, malayan
Brunn's syndrome in taeniasis 124

C

Calabar swellings in loiasis 82, 83
cancrum oris in visceral leishmaniasis 45, 47
Carrión's disease *see* bartonellosis
Casoni test in echinococcosis 116, 117
cestode infections 110–17, 122–6
Chagas' disease *see* American trypanosomiasis
chiclero ulcer in mucocutaneous leishmaniasis 54–5
Chickungunya fever 154, 159
Chilomastix mesnili 16
chloroquine
  ocular toxicity 176
  use in
    amoebiasis 26
    clonorchiasis 119
    malaria 11, 13, 179, 185
chlorpromazine, use in hyperpyrexia 179

cholera 136–42
  clinical features 139–40
  diagnosis 140
  distribution 136–7
  pathological features 137–9
  prevention 142 *and see* vaccination
  treatment 141–2
  vaccination 142, 186, 188
  'washerwoman's fingers' 139
Chopra's test in visceral leishmaniasis 47
chorioretinitis in
  onchoceriasis 79
  toxoplasmosis 58, 59, 60
Chrysops, vector in loiasis 82, 83
chyluria in filariasis 69–77 *passim*
clonorchiasis 118–19
Clyndamycin, use in toxoplasmosis 62
Councilman bodies in yellow fever 156
creeping eruption *see* larva migrans
Culex, vector in filariasis 68, 73, 77
cutaneous leishmaniasis 48–53
  clinical features 50
  diagnosis 50–2
  distribution 48
  pathological features 49–50
  table of characteristics 49
  treatment 52–3
cysts in
  amoebiasis 15–20, 26
  echinococcosis 111–16
  paragonimiasis 120–1
  taeniasis solium 124–5
  toxoplasmosis 57

D

deerfly see *Chrysops*
dengue and related fevers 156, 158–9
Desmonts' studies in toxoplasmosis 58
diamidodiphenol sulphone (DDS), use in leprosy 135–6
Dientamoeba fragilis 16
diethylcarbamazine (Hetrazan), use in
  filariasis 74, 77
  loiasis 83
  onchocerciasis 80
  tropical pulmonary eosinophilia 85
diethyltoluamide, insect repellent 85
Dipetalonema perstans, D. streptocerca 74
Diphyllobothrium latum infection 126
dracontiasis (dracunculosis) 84–5
Dupuytren contractures in yaws 162
dwarf tapeworm *see Hymenolepis nana*

E

echinococcosis 110–17
  alveolar hydatid disease 171
  clinical features 114–15
  cysts 111–16
  diagnosis 115–16
  distribution 110
  E. granulosus 111–13
  E. multilocularis 117
  'hydatid sand' 112
  'hydatid thrill 115
  treatment 116–17
egg morphology (illustrated)
  Ancylostoma duodenale 67
  Ascaris lumbricoides 89
  Clonorchus sinensis 118, 119
  Enterobius vermiculari. 87
  Heterophyes heterophyes 121
  Hymenolepis nana 125
  Necator americanus 67
  Paragonimus westermani 121
  Schistosoma haematobium 105, 106
  S. mansoni 100
  Taenia saginata, *T. solium* 123, 124
  Trichuris trichiura 92
elephantiasis *see* filariasis, bancroftian
El Tor vibrio in cholera 137
emetine hydrochloride, use in
  amoébiasis 24, 25, 26
encephalitis in arbor virus infections
  154, 158, 159
endarteritis in espundia 54
Endolimax nana 16
Entamoeba coli 16
E. histolytica see amoebiasis
entamide furoate, use in amoebiasis 26
enterobiasis 86–7
eosinophilia in
  ascariasis 118
  clonorchiasis 118
  echinococcosis 116
  larva migrans 94
  loiasis 83
  onchocerciasis 80
  paragonimiasis 121
  schistosomiasis 97, 101, 109
  strongyloidiasis 91
  taeniasis 122, 124
  trichiasis 93
  tropical pulmonary eosinophilia 85
epidemic typhus *see* rickettsioses
espundia *see* mucocutaneous
  leishmaniasis

F

Faget's sign in yellow fever and dengue
  156, 158
fasciolopsiasis 122
filariasis and related infections 68–85
  bancroftian 68–77
    chyluria *passim*
    clinical features 70–3
    diagnosis and treatment 73–7
    distribution and incidence 68
    elephantiasis *passim*
    microfilariae 69, 73–4
    pathological features 68–70
    Wuchereria bancrofti 68, 74
  malayan 77
  minor filarial infections 78–85
    dracontiasis (guinea worm disease)
      84–5
    loiasis *see separate entry*
    onchocerciasis *see separate entry*
Flagyl *see* metronidazole
flukes
  blood *see* schistosomiasis
  intestinal 121–2
  liver, Chinese and other 118–19
  lung 119–21
fluorescent antibody testing in
  African trypanosomiasis 34
  malaria 11
  toxoplasmosis 61
  visceral leishmaniasis 46
formal-gel test 46

G

Gammexane, insecticide 41
gangosa in yaws 162
gefilte fish and *D. latum* infection 126
Giardia lamblica 17, 27
giardiasis *see* amoebiasis
Glossina see African trypanosomiasis
Gnathostoma spinigerum in larva
  migrans 93
Guarnieri bodies in smallpox 147, 148
guinea worm *see* dracontiasis

H

Haemagogus, vector in yellow fever 153
haemoglobinopathies *see* tropical
  ophthalmology
halazone for water purification 189

Halberstaedter–Prowazek (H–P)
  bodies in trachoma 171
Hansen's bacillus in leprosy 127
heat, effects of 178–80
helminthic diseases 63–126
Herbert's pits in trachoma 171
heterophysiasis 121–2
Hetrazan *see* diethylcarbamazine
hexyresorcinol, use in
  fasciolopsiasis 122
Hippelates pallipes, vector in
  treponematoses 160, 164
Hippocratic facies in cholera 140
hookworm 63–8
  anaemia 64–5, 66, 68
  Ancylostoma duodenale 63–4, 66–8
  clinical features and diagnosis 66–7
  distribution and incidence 63
  Necator americanus 64, 66–7
  pathological features 63–6
  treatment 67–8
hydatid disease *see* echinococcosis
Hymenolepis nana 125
hyperpyrexia 179
hypovitaminosis A 174

I

Iodamoeba buetschlii 16
immunizations 185–8
  table of inoculations 186
  see also vaccination
insecticides, use in
  American trypanosomiasis 41
  leishmaniasis 48, 55
  malaria 1
  onchocerciasis 82
  personal protection 185
  rickettsioses 168, 188

J

Japanese B encephalitis 154, 158
jungle yellow fever 153

K

kala-azar *see* visceral leishmaniasis
Kedrowsky antigen in visceral
  leishmaniasis 46
Kerandel's sign in African
  trypanosomiasis 32
'kissing' bug *see* American
  trypanosomiasis

Kupffer's cells in
  malaria 9
  visceral leishmaniasis 43, 46
kuru 120–1
Kyasanur Forest virus 154, 158

L

larva migrans 93–4
Leishman–Donovan bodies 43
leishmaniasis *see* cutaneous leishmaniasis,
  mucocutaneous leishmaniasis,
  visceral leishmaniasis
leprosy 127–36
  clinical features 129–34
  diagnosis 134–5
  epidemiological aspects 128–9
  history 127
  lepra reaction 135
  lepromin test 134
  pathological features 129–34
  treatment 135–6
  types 128, 129
loiasis 82–3
  distribution 82
  eosinophilia 83
  microfilariae 82, 83
Lomidine *see* pentamidine isethionate

M

Machado–Guerreiro test in American
  trypanosomiasis 40
malaria 1–13
  blackwater fever 8, 11, 13
  clinical features 9–10
  diagnosis 10–11
  drugs and Plasmodium life cycle 12
  eradication schemes 1–2
  incidence 1
  pathological features 2–9
  pernicious forms 8
  prevention 13, 185
  treatment 11–13, 185
male fern, use in taeniasis 124
malnutrition and eye disease 174–5
Mansonella ozzardi 74
Mansonia, vector in malayan filariasis 77
Manson's schistosomiasis *see* S. *mansoni*
  infection
Maurer's clefts in falciparum malaria 2
meclazine hydrochloride 189
medical kit for the tropics 184

Mel B (Arsobal)
  ocular toxicity   177
  use in African trypanosomiasis   34
mepacrine *see* quinacrine hydrochloride
metagonimiasis   122
metronidazole (Flagyl), use in
  amoebiasis,25, 26
  giardiasis   27
  tropical ulcer   166
microfilariae   69, 73–4, 77, 78–9, 82, 83
milk precautions in tropics   189
Mitsuda–Rost reaction in leprosy   134
motion sickness   189
Mott, morular cells of   30
mucocutaneous leishmaniasis   48–9, 53–5
  diagnosis   55
  distribution   53–4
  espundia   54
  immunity   55
  treatment   55–6
  uta   55
Murray Valley virus   154, 158

N

Necator americanus see hookworm
nematode infections   63–94
niclosamide *see* Yomesan
niridazole (Ambilhar), use in
      schistosomiasis   102, 107, 109
N.N.N. media, use in
  American trypanosomiasis   40
  cutaneous leishmaniasis   51
  visceral leishmaniasis   46

O

onchocerciasis   78–82
  clinical features   79–80
  diagnosis   80
  distribution and incidence   78
  eosinophilia   79, 80
  eye lesions   79
  nodules   79, 80
  Onchocerca volvulus   78, 81
  pathological features   78–9
  treatment   80–2
Onyong-nyong fever   154, 159
Oriental schistosomiasis *see*
      S. japonicum infection
Oroya fever *see* bartonellosis

P

paragonimiasis   119–21
Paschen bodies in smallpox   147
Pasteurella pestis   143
pentamidine isethionate, use in African
      trypanosomiasis   34
Pfeiffer phenomenon in cholera   137
Phlebotomus, vector in bartonellosis   145
  leishmaniasis   42, 49, 53, 55
  sandfly fever   159
pinworm *see* enterobiasis
pinta   164–5
piperazine, use of, in
  ascariasis   90
  enterobiasis   87
plague   142–4
pork tapeworm *see* Taeniasis solium
post-kala-azar dermal leishmaniasis   45
primaquine, use of, in malaria   11, 185
protozoal diseases   1–62
pyrimethane, use of, in toxoplasmosis
      61–2

Q

Q fever *see* rickettsioses
quinacrine hydrochloride, use of, in
  cutaneous leishmaniasis   32
  giardiasis   27
quinine and malaria   11–13
  ocular toxicity   176

R

reduviid bugs of *Triatoma*   35, 36, 38
'rice-water' stools in cholera   137, 138
rickettsioses   166–9
  table of types   167
Rift Valley fever   154, 159
Romaña's sign in American
      trypanosomiasis   37, 38

S

Sabin–Feldman test in toxoplasmosis   61
sandfly *see Phlebotomus*
sandfly fever   154, 159
schistosomiasis   94–110
  rare schistosomal infections   110
  Schistosoma haematobium infections
      (bilharziasis, urinary
      schistosomiasis)   103–7

schistosomiasis—*continued*
   clinical features 104–5
   diagnosis 105
   distribution and incidence 103
   pathological features 103–4
   protection 190
   treatment 107
  S. japonicum infections 107–10
   clinical features 108
   diagnosis 108–9
   distribution and incidence 107–8
   pathological features 108
   treatment 109–10
  S. mansoni infections 94–103
   clinical features 98–9
   diagnosis 100–1
   distribution and incidence 94–5
   pathological features 95–8
   treatment 101–2
schizonts in malaria 2–12
Schüffner's dots in malaria 2, 3, 6
scrub typhus *see* rickettsioses
Simulium, vector in
  onchocerciasis 78, 80
  pinta 164
sleeping sickness, East African, Gambian,
   Rhodesian, West African *see*
   African trypanosomiasis
smallpox 146–52
  clinical features 147, 149–50
  diagnosis 150
  incidence 146
  pathological features 146–7, 148
  treatment 151
  vaccination 146, 151–2, 185–7
sparganosis *see* tropical ophthalmology
Spiramycin, use in toxoplasmosis 61, 62
spotted fevers *see* rickettsioses
Stoll count in hookworm 66
strongyloidiasis 91–2
suramin (Antrypol), use in
  African trypanosomiasis 34
  onchocerciasis 80

T

taeniasis saginata 122–4
taeniasis solium 124–5
tapeworm *see* taeniasis,
   Diphyllobothrium latum,
   Hymenolepis nana
tapir nose in leishmaniasis 54
tartar emetic, use in schistosomiasis 109
tetrachlorethylene, use in

heterophysiasis 122
hookworm 67
metagonimiasis 122
thiabendazole, use in
  dracontiasis 85
  larva migrans 93
  strongyloidiasis 92
  trichiasis 93
  trichinosis 91
Toxocara canis in larva migrans 94
toxoplasmosis 56–62
  clinical features and diagnosis 58–61
  distribution 56–7
  iatrogenic factors 56
  ocular infections 56, 59, 60, 62
  pathological features 57–8
  treatment and prevention 61–2
trachoma 170–3
  Arlt's lines 173
  diagnosis 171, 173
  Halberstaedter–Prowazek (H–P)
   bodies 171
  Herbert's pits 171
  incidence 170
  treatment 171
trematode infections 94–110, 117–22
trench fever *see* rickettsioses
treponematoses 160–6
  pinta 164
  tropical ulcer (TPU) 165–6
  yaws 160–3
Triatoma see African trypanosomiasis
trichiasis 92–3
trichinosis 90–1
Trichomonas hominis 17
tropical ophthalmology 170–7
  haemoglobinopathies 175
  iatrogenic factors 175–6
  mechanical factors 177
  sparganosis 171–4
  trachoma *see separate entry*
tropical pulmonary eosinophilia (T.P.E.)
   85
tropical sprue 181–2
tropical travel advice 183–90
  before departure 183–6
  en route 188–9
  immunizations 186–8
  in the tropics 189–90
  on return 190
tropical ulcer *see* treponematoses
trypanosomiasis *see* African, American
   trypanosomiasis
tryparsamide 34, 176
tsetse fly *see* African trypanosomiasis
typhus *see* rickettsioses

U

Uganda S virus 154, 158, 159
Uncinaria stenocephala in larva migrans
  93
urinary schistosomiasis *see*
  schistosomiasis, *S. haematobium*
uta *see* mucocutaneous leishmaniasis

V

vaccination for
  cholera 142, 186, 188
  diphtheria 186, 187
  hepatitis 186, 188
  plague 186, 188
  tetanus 186, 187
  typhoid 186, 187
  typhus 168, 186, 188
  yellow fever 157–8, 186, 187–8
varicella differentiated from smallpox
  149–50
variola *see* smallpox
Venezuelan encephalitis 159
verruga peruana in bartonellosis 145
viral diseases 146–59
visceral leishmaniasis (kala–azar) 42–8
  'black fever' 44
  clinical features 43–5
  diagnosis 42–3
  distribution and incidence 42
  leishmanin skin test, 46, 47
  pathological features 42–3
  post-kala-azar dermal form 45
  prevention 48
  serum proteins 43
  table of types and characteristics 44
  treatment 48

W

'washerwoman's fingers' in cholera 139
Wassermann false reaction 30

water precautions in tropics 188, 189
Weil–Felix reaction in rickettsioses 168
West Nile fever 154, 158, 159
whipworm *see* trichiasis
Winterbottom's sign in African
  trypanosomiasis 32
Wolbach's nodules in rickettsioses 167
Wuchereria bancrofti see filariasis

X

xenodiagnosis in American
  trypanosomiasis 40
Xenophylla cheopsis, vector in plague 143

Y

yaws 160–4
  bejel and other local names 160, 163
  early lesions 160–2
  intermediate forms 163–4
  late lesions 162–3
  transmission 160
  treatment 164
yellow fever 152–8
  clinical features 156
  diagnosis 156–7
  distribution 152–3
  epidemiology 153–4
  pathological features 156–7
  treatment 157–8
  vaccination 157–8, 186, 187–8
Yomesan (niclosamide), use in cestode
  infections 123, 125, 126

Z

Ziemann's dots in malaria 2
Z-plasty, use in ainhum 181